No Longer A SECRET

Unique Common Sense Strategies for

Children with Sensory or Motor Challenges

D1566201

Doreit Sarah Bialer, MA, OTR/L

Lucy Jane Miller, PhD, OTR

No Longer A SECRET:

Unique Common Sense Strategies for Children with Sensory or Motor Challenges

All marketing and publishing rights guaranteed to and reserved by:

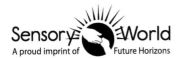

1010 N. Davis Drive
Arlington, Texas 76012
(877) 775-8968
(682) 558-8941
(682) 558-8945 (fax)
E-mail: *info@sensoryworld.com*
www.sensoryworld.com

Cover and interior design, Cindy Williams

ISBN: 9781935567295

Dedication

I dedicate this book to both of my children, Arianna Rachel and Alec Ross. You both inspire me to continue my journey in helping children and families with Sensory Processing Disorder. Many special thanks to my sister, Zipora, and to my mom, for your unconditional love and support, and to Annie, Anthony, and Keri for believing in me.

~ *D. S. B.*

To the children, mothers and fathers, and siblings who have been my "professors" on this journey to understanding Sensory Processing Disorder. Special thanks to my colleague, Dr Sarah A. Schoen, who joined our team a decade ago and has made countless contributions to developing our dream. And to my staff at the STAR Center and the Sensory Processing Disorder Foundation: None of this would have happened without your generosity and dedication, above and beyond what anyone could expect. It does, after all, take a village to provide hope and help to children with SPD and their families.

To our readers: We look forward to seeing each and every one of you, either as clients at the STAR Center or in our advanced mentorships at the Sensory Processing Disorder Foundation!

~ *L.J.M.*

Table of Contents

Preface

◆

Doreit's Story

It wasn't until I adopted my first child that I'd ever loved anyone so intensely that no words could describe the feeling. I remember the phone call we got to congratulate my husband and me for being the "new adoptive parents" of our son, born in February 1995. We were both so overjoyed, we screamed and cried—it was a mixture of a thousand emotions that had been pent up for so long.

Our precious boy, Alec Ross, awaited our arrival 9 days after his birth. The delay in bringing him home from the hospital stemmed from "a couple of minor concerns"—he was jaundiced and had a small head. Still, we were assured that he was perfect. My best friend at the time, a neonatologist, carefully read all the medical reports and asked if we were sure we wanted to go through with this particular adoption. "Are you kidding?" my husband and I answered. "Of course!" And so we began our personal education in Sensory Processing Disorder (SPD).

Our son came home from the hospital with projectile vomiting and severe irritability. Among many distressing behaviors, Alec fought against being held and kissed. As a new mom, I was at once madly in love but stressed out and confused. By the time he was 15 days old, I'd arranged for an early-intervention team to start evaluating our son, who cried throughout their assessment. After what seemed like a lifetime, the therapists left and came back with a caseworker within a week's time. My husband and I were presented with a long list of our son's problems. My mind wandered as I blocked out the therapists' presentation. It sounded like a lot of noise to me. Their words were impersonal and offered no solutions—the team just went through a long list of worries that seemed to rationalize the need for each of their intensive intervention services. In all their chatter, I remember looking down at my sleeping baby and thinking, "These people don't really know you." And you know what? I was right.

◆

That team of professionals, confabbing in our living room 16 years ago, knew nothing at all about Alec Ross. They knew nothing about how well he would ice skate at age 5 or how much he'd love tinkering with engines when he was 11. They had no idea how creative and artistic he would become. They couldn't predict how easily he'd be able to say "I love you" as a teenager, and really mean it. And they couldn't have known that he would grow up to be one of the most tender young men on the planet. To them, Alec was just a cluster of challenges and symptoms. Still, we needed their help. "Thank you all," I remember telling the therapists, as they handed me a long list of expensive therapy equipment to buy and a schedule of dates and times they'd be coming back to work with my son.

Until you experience being the parent of a child with SPD, you can't really understand the desperation of wanting to help, the vulnerability to experts' advice, and the willingness to do whatever is necessary at whatever cost— even if it means turning your warm and cozy home into a therapy clinic. No treatment is too expensive, no intervention is too time-consuming, and no doctor's office is too far if it means potentially sparing your child the negative feedback, social awkwardness, name-calling, isolation, confusion, and low self-esteem that come with SPD. What's essential is to remember who your sensational child is, beyond labels and diagnoses. He or she has beautiful and amazing talents that maybe only you get to see. Alec is not only a kid with sensory craving and dyspraxia. He's a smart, funny, polite, talented, personable, charming, and passionate 16-year-old who has lots of dreams that keep him going. Always knowing that—even during the loudest tantrums and toughest meltdowns—has helped our family navigate our way through it.

Professionally, my education in SPD started 15 years into my career as an occupational therapist, when the school where I was working asked me to greet students at the bus every morning. Immediately, I noticed remarkable differences in the way the children got off the bus. Some kids jumped down the stairs and skipped to the classroom, where they eagerly unpacked their belongings and got ready to start their day. Others had to be carried off the bus, screaming and kicking. It was clear that these differences seemed to reflect more than the kids' attitudes about school. The bus ride itself, I realized, could be overwhelming. The bumps and noises, the stops and starts, the close contact with other kids, and the invasion of personal space could be completely overloading and disorganizing to some children. Why, I wondered, could some kids cope on the bus, while others fell apart?

As it turned out, many of the kids who had trouble staying seated on their 30-minute ride to school also couldn't sit still during math lessons. It wasn't a coincidence that the first-grader who found the bus ride too noisy in the mornings cowered from the drumming in music class each afternoon. And it was no wonder that the third-grader who panicked whenever anyone opened a window on the bus also lost concentration when his teacher turned on a fan to cool down the classroom. Children like these were clearly experiencing sensory input differently than their schoolmates. They were demonstrating signs of SPD—the patterns were obvious.

My personal experiences with my son and professional experiences in helping students cope with their own sensory challenges led me to devise strategies and low-cost tools to assist kids with SPD. In time, I came to learn that kids don't need fancy therapy equipment or brand names to deal with sensorimotor challenges. Just as nobody's jump shot improves by buying a pair of LeBron James Nikes, the nervous system doesn't care what brand of therapy equipment you use or how much it costs.

In the schools where I worked, special services never had the budgets to buy much gear at all. It was up to me to bring my own equipment to treat children who qualified for occupational-therapy services. The more my caseload grew, the more I bought. Eventually, I lugged my menagerie of equipment to school each day in a rolling suitcase. Soon, my role as an occupational therapist began to change as teachers asked for more and more help in the classroom. It became unrealistic to walk up and down flights of stairs with a heavy Samsonite. Besides, students were facing so many different issues in each classroom that the concept of "one size fits all" wasn't going to work.

That's when I started making individualized, low-tech objects for each child. This required spontaneity and creativity in using items readily available in the classroom. My favorite ones included a 2-inch loose-leaf binder, enlarged rubber bands, masking tape, and students' own jackets and sweaters. With these, I found ways of developing substitutes for therapeutic items, including wedges for posture, slant boards, sitting disks, bolsters, balance boards, weighted vests, compression jackets, and even suspended equipment. I realized that my students didn't recognize the differences or care about whether we were using expensive, "state-of-the-art" equipment from the glossy catalogues. In fact, most of the kids beyond first grade were happy to learn strategies based on materials that didn't look different or "weird."

Remembering how important it is to establish relationships and trust with kids, I got so adept at making positive changes without all the fancy stuff that I finally left my suitcase behind. When the economy faltered in 2008, using everyday objects became even more imperative to the families of students, to the schools, and to my own practice. I let everyone know that we would figure out how to meet each child's needs by making our own substitutes to replace pricy, brand-named equipment.

In 2010, I registered for an intensive mentorship program at the Sensory Processing Disorder Foundation in Colorado, which was taught by Dr Lucy Jane Miller, Dr Sarah Schoen, and staff members of the Sensory Therapies And Research (STAR) Center, which Dr Miller directs. It was a life-changing experience. I shared my ideas with Dr Miller, and we decided to coauthor this book to build on my experiences with low-cost, low-tech strategies to help children with SPD. Writing this book has been a meaningful journey for me, and one that I hope you will learn from. Most of all, I want to convey hope to all parents—that you can help your kids by using thoughtful strategies that do not involve expensive, technologically sophisticated equipment. As Dr Miller always says, "The best tool you have to help a child with SPD is *you!*"

We urge you to review the chapters in consecutive order and not skip around on the assumption that one particular subtype of SPD pertains to your child. Children with SPD usually don't fit neatly into a single classification. They typically demonstrate behaviors indicative of issues in more than one subtype. So please stay with it—all of it. Take the time to learn about all of the many aspects of the disorder—the subtypes and the symptoms. Learn how to use Dr Miller's strategic approach, which she dubs "A SECRET." SPD treatment does not need to be perplexing and expensive any longer.

Doreit Sarah Bialer

April 2011

Thoughts from Lucy Jane Miller

What happens when something feels bad, but you don't know what's wrong with you? How are you supposed to feel when your condition has been diagnosed, then rediagnosed, and you don't understand any of it? Where do you go when you feel lost and confused, when no one believes you and not even your parents know what to do?

As a teenager, I had a serious problem. I was losing my eyesight, and no one could figure out why. I could see with my contact lenses, but when I took them out, images were fuzzy and diffuse. Things got worse over time, and by the age of 15, I could barely detect anything except light and dark without my contacts. The lenses hurt my eyes, and I'd often blink one out and have to spend hours on my hands and knees trying to find it. I'd had a happy childhood until I "went weird" as a teenager.

My parents—who were both loving, educated professionals—took me to an ophthalmologist, who said there was nothing wrong with my eyes. "It's all in her head," he said. On some level, pretty much everyone suspected I was making up the blurriness, the pain of wearing contacts—the whole deal. My pediatrician and school nurse were sure I'd scripted this teenage drama to get attention. My high-school guidance counselor knew about this psychiatric issue of Lucy "making things up" and advised me not to apply to a top-tier college, saying, "Go where you know you'll be accepted, Lucy, or you may not get in at all."

Even I, myself, began to wonder what could be so wrong in my head that I was imagining all these eye issues. I thought maybe I was crazy. And if I was, what could I do about it? I was still a child. Where could I turn? In that era, the 1960s, *psychiatrist* was a word that conjured up mental institutions, shock therapy, and people roaming the grounds, foaming at the mouth. I felt alone with my fuzzy vision and fears.

What happened next is laid out in my first book, *Sensational Kids*, but what's key to the book you're reading now are two painful memories. One was that *people didn't believe me*. To this day, that has affected and shaped my life. The other was that my sensations *weren't like* those of my friends. Although I saw less, I heard much more (my children claim I can hear through walls!). And I *felt* more, both through my fingertips and through my heart and soul. This became apparent in my early 20s, when I finally received a diagnosis of keratoconus and was treated by receiving corneal transplants. After the transplant surgeries, both my eyes were patched for 6 months, and I wasn't allowed to move my body or head. During that time, I noticed that when somebody walked into my room, I'd know immediately how he or she was feeling, even if the person was a stranger. As "woo-woo" as that may seem, it's true. As palpably as any sight, sound, or smell, I could tell if a person was happy, angry, embarrassed, or whatever. I could sense how people were feeling.

This intense awareness of my own shifting sensory boundaries prompted me to spend the next 35 years studying children's sensory systems and trying to help parents and siblings understand *sensational* kids. In many ways, my work—like that of many professionals in the "helping" professions—is an attempt to work out the frustrations and anxieties I experienced during my own youth.

Lots of folks don't believe in SPD. As you can imagine, that makes research very difficult. The National Institutes of Health (NIH) (which funds most health research in the United States) doesn't look fondly on funding disorders that "don't exist." SPD won't become "official" in the eyes of the NIH until rigorous research allows us to characterize the disorder, identify its genetic and environmental causes, demonstrate the parts of the brain that are disrupted, and prove that the symptoms are continuous in a single person from infancy through school age and beyond. Without these data, the condition isn't "real," and if it's not *really* a disorder, you can't get funding to study it. Without funding, however, you can't verify whether or not it's a valid disorder. Does anybody else notice the catch-22 here?

So what now?

We must work locally and globally to build our awareness, so that all people—children and adults alike—who struggle with sensory-processing problems get what they need to cope: early identification, assessment, and treatment, if needed.

This book follows up on many ideas launched in *Sensational Kids,* which tells the story of five children with SPD as they proceed through a typical day. The purpose of that book was to explain the primary types of the disorder in a way that a reader could relate to and understand. Although it touched on intervention, there wasn't enough space to really explain treatment. Treatment for SPD is complex, as is diagnosis of the disorder. All too often, neither assessment nor treatment is done well. It takes a seasoned therapist (usually an occupational therapist) who has experience *and* has received guidance from an even more experienced therapist to be able to understand the nuances of the assessment of SPD. Advanced mentorship is needed to diagnose SPD accurately.

Learning to treat by using the best processes known today brings a completely different set of learning needs on the part of the provider of service. If you've ever looked through a one-way mirror at therapy session with a clinician— usually an occupational therapist—it may seem that the child and therapist are "just playing," but in actuality the therapist is providing individualized, play-based treatment that continually challenges the child to succeed. Ah, the joy of mastery…it can only be experienced after the intensive effort that a "just-right-challenge" provides. The child moves forward with challenge…then success. Next comes a harder challenge…then success again. And so on. This constitutes the cycle of effective, intuitive treatment.

After years of observing, consulting, and running the mentorship program for experienced therapists at the STAR Center and the SPD Foundation (co-directed by Dr Sarah A. Schoen, my dedicated teaching partner and close friend), I'm well aware of therapists who are trained in a traditional model of treating sensory issues who are feeling dissatisfied and "stuck." Having been trained and mentored by Dr A. Jean Ayres in a 12-week mentorship in which we trained 5 days per week, I too used her treatment model for decades. In fact, the randomized clinical trial that my colleagues and I published in 2007 was a 15-year culmination of research that provided empirical evidence for the validity of this approach.[1] Although the Ayres Sensory Integration treatment approach is incredibly valuable and effective with certain children, I've become convinced that other aspects of intervention are equally important. Regulating a child's arousal levels, for example, deserves more emphasis in treatment. So, too, do elements of relationships and engagement, processing auditory stimulation, developing cognitive behavioral strategies, and certainly fostering parent education and coaching.

Doreit Bialer asked for my feedback on an early version of this manuscript during her mentorship program at the Sensory Processing Disorder Foundation/STAR Center. Her approaches appealed to me. I loved the idea of implementing low-cost, low-tech strategies for children with sensorimotor issues. I also wanted to help a wider audience understand the underlying principles trained experts use to treat their young clients and learn to problem-solve on their own.

In Doreit, I discovered an open-minded and enthusiastic collaborator who was delighted to organize her manuscript into the subtypes my colleagues and I proposed[2] and to use the treatment framework (called "A SECRET") from *Sensational Kids*.

Together, we've written this book for you. At times, we speak directly to you, the parents. Other times, we speak to you, the teachers. And at points we speak to you, the therapists. We all have so much to learn. I often say, "The kids are *my* professors." When a child is particularly complex or puzzling, he or she becomes our best teacher of all. We don't know exactly why occupational therapy works. We must be humble about what we know and openly admit what we don't know. And we must continue to grow by asking questions every day.

Though the research is ever-evolving,[3] I do know this much for certain: SPD is not a reflection of bad behavior, and it is not caused by bad parenting. In fact, it's not "bad" at all. It's physiologic in nature.

If you are worried that your child might have SPD, take the first step and get an evaluation by a multidisciplinary team. (For more information on multidisciplinary evaluations, go to *www.STARCenter.us/Sensory-Processing-Assessment-Treatment-Therapy.html*.) You can also join (or start) your local SPD Parent Connections group. The earlier the right subtype of SPD is diagnosed, the earlier a child will learn to cope with it. And the sooner parents learn "A SECRET" when it comes to helping their son or daughter, the sooner stresses will ease in the whole family. I do not mean that parents should become therapists. Instead, families should be taught the *principles* of therapy, rather than just trying to follow their therapist's suggestions. Then families and therapists can work together to embed therapeutic interventions into the natural day of children who are receiving treatment.

We hope this book gives you a framework for strategies to use the next time you need them. There is help. There is hope. We're all in this together. And, believe me—no matter what the doubts of the medical orthodoxy—there are a lot of us.

Dr Lucy Jane Miller

April 2011

A Letter to Parents

To our Parent Partners—

We've written this book for you—our greatest source of inspiration and our most important audience. Every day we work with parents like you, the hidden heroes and heroines of this journey, who make the lives of children with Sensory Processing Disorder (SPD) as happy and fulfilling as possible.

Children learn the most important things in life from you, their parents—how to love, play, negotiate, compromise, win graciously, and lose with equanimity. Kids learn what being a good sibling means. They learn how to be helped and supported, how to help others, and how to support those less able than themselves. And, they learn that they have unlimited potential, as long as they recognize and adapt to their areas of challenge. These lessons have nothing to do with therapy protocols, such as how to tolerate a brushing program, when to wear a weighted vest, or how to incorporate heavy work.

Many of the children who come to us at the Sensory Therapies and Research (STAR) Center have been through multiple evaluations and at least a few therapeutic programs. Although some of those therapy experiences have been helpful, parents often feel obliged to "follow through" with therapeutic protocols at home and sometimes at school, as well. Our message to parents is this: "You are a *parent first*. Therapy programs should be devised with your schedule in mind. You are *not* a surrogate therapist."

In fact, your job as a parent isn't prescriptive. It has nothing to do with making sure your child sucks thick applesauce through a straw or spends enough time in positions that defy gravity. Your main job is to be loving, positive, fun, supportive, and rewarding toward your child and to create magical moments during which you laugh together, hang out, and spend time together.

"But, how?" you may ask. "There is so much therapy I have to do to follow up...I want the best for my child." And the answer is simple yet fundamental: *Playing with your child is crucially important and should be your first priority.* I always ask parents at the STAR Center how many hours a week they play with their child, and, often, the answer sounds something like, "We do the [whatever type of protocol] every day. We do occupational therapy twice a week, speech therapy three times a week, therapeutic horseback riding on Saturdays, and adaptive gymnastics on Tuesday nights."

"Great!" I say. "I can see you are doing everything you possibly can to help Nellie. But how many hours a week do you just *play* with Nellie?"

This book contains a lot of information—too much to take in on one reading! But if you only get *one key message* from this book, it is this: *Enjoy your child. Spend time down on the floor pretending to be bugs, out in the yard tossing a ball, in the family room acting out imaginary figures, or dressing up as favorite characters. Through this simple act, your child will learn the most important lessons in life and will feel treasured and important.*

There are children who are winners and, on the other side, children who eventually lose their natural joy and spontaneity and struggle to live satisfying lives. My personal experience is that if a child thinks he or she is a *great kid* by second grade, that kid will grow up to become a *great adult*. Children who feel that they are somehow "bad" or that there are big things "wrong" with them by the second grade have a hard time overcoming feelings of inadequacy and can often make foolish choices as teenagers and adults, resulting in lost opportunities and potential.

My recipe for therapy time versus play is this: Spend at least as many hours playing with your child as you do in therapy (including the drive to and from the session). Two hours of therapy a week + ½ hour each way in the car (1 hour x 2 sessions) is 4 hours a week total. For that level of therapeutic intervention, then, a child should play with his mom or dad for 4 or more hours per week.

"But," you say, "I thought getting therapy is what my child needed." While therapy is a way to help kids become more comfortable in areas of challenge, these areas should not define them. Without the proper balance between therapy and play, the message kids get is that they need "fixing." Play helps them intrinsically understand all the ways in which they are great kids. It sends an important message that parents, siblings, and friends think they are special, valued, and loved.

"But what do you mean *'play'?"* one dad asked me. "I don't understand what you mean. Is there a book I can read about that?"

All you really need to remember is what it's like to "just play," like when you were a kid—without agenda and without structure. We as a society have become entirely too purpose-driven in our children's activities. After school, kids are driven to soccer practice, piano lessons, or art classes. Many children start school early so they can fit Spanish lessons in. But how many kids just "hang out," riding their bikes with their buddies? How many 6- to 9-year-olds are out in their yards, pretending to be pirates or cowboys or Jedi warriors? When is the last time you saw a child look for a scarf to use as a pretend mask/ magic vest/transporter? Or do a made-up dance? Or give you handmade tickets for a play staged with the neighbors down the street?

This is what all our kids need—the freedom to play and make up their own games. Time to negotiate rules with their play partners. Time to try. Time to succeed. And time to learn from less-than-successful ventures. And where does the platform for the rules for play come from? It comes from their interactions with you when you are playing with them. For many typically developing children, this happens at a very young age; but for our *sensational kids*, it comes when they are emotionally ready, which may be many years past when typically developing children learn these rules of engagement.

Do I believe in therapy? Of course I do! I have devoted my life to research, education, and advocacy for SPD. I direct a therapeutic clinic, the STAR Center, where we help hundreds of kids and their families. But, we help them by empowering parents to know what to do for their own child. We empower them through parent education and coaching (parents are usually a part of therapy sessions). We empower them by reframing "bad" behaviors as physiologic needs rather than as willful obstruction and power struggles.

Our job as your child's occupational therapist or other professional supporter isn't to be your friend, your personal support system, your child's companion, or a referee for family strife. It is to teach you to know enough about your child that you can help him or her cope with sensory challenges whenever and wherever they occur. It's to train you to think ahead and strategize, so problems are less likely to occur and so that you can problem-solve *in the moment* when problems do occur. We want you to feel self-assured and confident that *you* know how to do the best that can be done for your child.

This book is a tribute to your potential as a mom or dad to help your child more than any trained, licensed professional ever could. It's an affirmation of your ability to understand sensorimotor challenges. And it's a celebration of spending time with your child and being present as you figure out strategies to overcome those challenges together. As a therapist, it's my life's work to empower you as parents to know that you—and only you—are in charge of deciding what support mechanisms and services your child needs. And as a parent, it's your life's work to empower your *sensational kids*.

In writing this book, we didn't put in list after list of activities you should do. Instead, we have tried to show you how to think about—or *problem solve*—what might benefit your child most in a specific situation, given the challenges he or she has. Most of all, we want you to feel comfortable being a mom or a dad, a grandma, or an aunt. You don't need to know every little technical detail to help your child. You are better off knowing the *questions to ask* to get your child to the next point and through the tough times, than knowing a thousand therapeutic activities.

As a young therapist, my first mentor, Dr A. Jean Ayres, told me, "Lucy, learn to ask the questions. Focus on the questions—not the answers. If you ask the right questions, you'll learn the right answers." And so, I pass this wisdom on to you. Ask questions. Learn about the process and the concepts—do not focus on specific activities. You will grow, and your child will grow along with you. After all, you are a team—you and your whole family—and we are your consultants, who you allow into your life for a moment in time. We thank you for trusting us with your child and your concerns.

Finally, through this book, we want to hopefully leave you with two gifts… hope and help. They are there, somewhere, waiting for you to find them. Go out and get what you need, and make sure whomever you find to help you educates you to provide what your child needs. We're here to help you and to empower you to ask and answer your own questions about what needs to be tried next. After all, this support is what enables you to be confident and remain positive.

Remember—laugh, giggle, have fun, and focus on *joie de vivre,* or "joy in life." That is the most important thing.

~ L. J. M.

A Letter to Teachers

Dear Teachers—

The role of the classroom teacher has become ever more challenging and difficult as the demands for "mainstreaming and inclusion" continue to grow. Teachers with thorough backgrounds in regular education are now expected to ensure that their classrooms meet the needs of all children. In many states, all children must meet mandatory academic state requirements, and the curriculum must be flexible enough to meet the diversified learning needs of all children.

The composition of learning styles in the regular public school classroom is even more complex than it was when only typically developing children were included. Now it is likely that in any particular classroom, you may find children with autism, Tourette syndrome, pervasive developmental delay, attention-deficit/hyperactivity disorder, SPD, and many other diagnoses. Regardless of the conditions involved, the biggest challenge for the classroom teacher is the varying degrees to which sensation, emotion, and attention affect the children in the classroom.

For learning to take place, children need predictable environments and tasks that are hard but at which they can succeed. The consequences of poor attention, abnormal arousal, and emotional regulation problems negatively affect learning, not just for the individual child manifesting the difficulty, but also for the whole class.

In this book, our goal is to provide you, the teacher, with a framework to develop your own tools for your classroom to help children in need of additional support to grow and learn. We use A SECRET framework to explain how to meet the sensory needs of children in your classroom for several reasons. Foremost, teachers are sometimes led to believe that the ideas therapists come up with are "secret" and take many years of study to learn. To some extent this is true, but what we have done in this book is help explain the *thinking process* that a therapist uses in devising a strategy for a particular student with sensory needs. We believe that once you know the process, there is no longer "a secret," at least not from you!

Teachers are the backbone of the future of our country. As K. Patricia Cross (a renowned social scientist who studied education) so aptly noted, "The task of the excellent teacher is to stimulate 'apparently ordinary' people to unusual effort. The tough problem is not in identifying winners—it is in making winners out of ordinary people."[4] And we would add to that… "In making winners out of all children—gifted, typically developing, and challenged." True teachers know that it is not the number of facts that really matters, it's the sense of mastery, of success, that matters in the long run for the children they teach.

We hope that understanding the SPD subtypes and the seven elements of A SECRET will expand your perspective as a teacher. We discuss the thinking process of devising modifications for children who need increased attention to their sensory needs to be successful learners in the classroom. Remember that by creating strategies that have just the right level of difficulty, you can help a child feel better about him- or herself. If you can enhance a challenged child's desire and success when participating with other children, you will have accomplished a huge and crucial task.

In some ways, who you are as a teacher is more important than what you teach in your classroom. In this book, we talk about regulating children and sharing your "inner self" with them so that overresponsive children become less aroused, underresponsive children wake up and become involved, and sensory cravers begin to find appropriate sensations to soothe their cravings. A good teacher lightens the burden of a child who knows that other children think he or she is different. Perhaps even more important is that an understanding teacher can guide parents toward a necessary evaluation and/or treatment without making a parent feel that something is "wrong" with their child.

In my life, next to my parents, my special teachers who made me feel talented and successful are the people who influenced me most—more than any textbook I read. The appreciation of a teacher can raise whatever you do from the mundane to the exceptional. I have been privileged to attend good schools and learn from some of the best educators. But I would not be who I am if it were not for the support of key teachers along the way…educators who told me that I could do it. Yes, it was hard, and yes, it might come easier to others, but I knew I could do whatever I wanted to do and that I could make a difference.

We hope more than anything that this book empowers you, our teachers, to feel that you can make a difference for children with sensory challenges.

We need you on the team. In fact, for some children, you will be the most important person on their team!

> One looks back with appreciation to the brilliant teachers, but with gratitude to those who touched our human feelings. The curriculum is so much necessary raw material, but warmth is the vital element for the growing plant and for the soul of the child.
>
> ~Carl Jung

~ *D. S. B.*

The Eight Sensory Systems, Sensory Processing, and SPD

Who Needs to Know What?

Some months ago, I was sitting in my office, waiting for the Janssens to arrive. They had been referred to me by the psychologist and the occupational therapist at the Sensory Therapies And Research (STAR) Center. Sophie and Cyril Janssen arrived out of breath, looking worried. I invited them to have a seat, and my assistant Caraly gave them each a glass of cold water. (I wished I had a sedative to offer them instead!)

"Well, what can I do for you?" I asked. "Can I answer any questions or clarify anything?"

"Yes," said Sophie, pulling out the four-page list she and Cyril had made. "My son Anthony has Sensory Processing Disorder. His nystagmus is abnormal, and his proprioceptive and vestibular systems are underresponsive. We've been told that his problem is probably cerebellar, and we've been working on that at home." (They were from Northern Maine.) "But, we've been here three days already, and we haven't seen any of our usual protocols, so we're afraid the occupational therapist is working on the wrong things with Anthony."

Wow! This evident confusion certainly explained part of Anthony's problems. It seemed that everyone around him was trying to attribute his behaviors to specific "affected" areas of the brain, as if they could treat individual areas of brain functioning. Obviously, Sophie and Cyril had learned this information from their occupational therapist. But for what purpose? How could hypothesizing about the *type* of brain dysfunction Anthony had help in treating his problems? Did the Janssens really understand the information they'd been given about the cerebellar, vestibular, and proprioceptive problems that Anthony supposedly had? Well, maybe they were physicians, I thought. I glanced down at their intake paperwork: *Mother (Sophie), CEO of a Fortune-500 company; Father (Cyril), physicist.* Did the anatomical matters we were dealing with really make sense to them in terms of helping Anthony?

"I understand," I said, in my most empathetic voice. "So what behaviors have you been working on?"

"We've been trying to correct all his sensory processing issues," Cyril answered. "He has so many problems, I don't even know where to begin. That's why we came all the way to Colorado, and we haven't seen anything good come out of it yet." (Remember—this was day 3.)

"Yes," Sophie jumped in. "We read about your neuroimaging studies, and that's what we want to get for Anthony, so we can find out what else is going on in his brain. Then we can work on that too, besides dealing with the cerebellar dysfunction."

My real purpose in sharing this story is to point out that occupational therapists who administer sensory-based therapy often go beyond the limits of their real area of knowledge in leading parents to think that we can diagnose dysfunction in specific areas of the brain. If this is, in fact, what we are doing when we report our clinical findings to parents, we are fooling not only them, but also ourselves.

When it comes to "neurological talk," occupational therapists need to understand that neuroscientists, neurologists, psychiatrists, and pediatricians have so much more training in the area of brain functioning than we do. At least most of them *know* what they don't know…and they would *never* go so far as to suggest verbally or in writing that a child has a vestibular problem without conducting neuroimaging or functional magnetic resonance imaging studies to show functional and structural brain evidence to support their statements.

In my experience, occupational therapists love to "talk neuro." That's fine in the office, when I'm surrounded by a group of enthusiastic occupational therapists who are just trying to understand what might be going on with a particular child. But what could be the point of leading the Janssens to think that Anthony had cerebellar problems, when they were not able to articulate a single, observable, functional goal? In this book, we do sometimes touch on neurological theories; but these are always identified with the qualifiers "as we suppose," or "perhaps," or "this might suggest," so you can differentiate hypotheses from the facts.

Occupational therapists know so much more than "neuro." When it comes to Sensory Processing Disorder (SPD), it would behoove us to admit that neuroanatomy really isn't our area of expertise. It's a shame that we feel compelled to "talk neuro" and perhaps convey information to parents that is neither accurate nor useful. As an occupational therapist, it takes very little time for us to assess why a child in a particular environment may feel unsuccessful and challenged. We can quickly come up with great strategies and suggestions for parents and teachers about how to make modifications that can help a child cope and feel more successful. That's what we are so skilled at doing! We have a tremendous gift when it comes to helping children. We need to realize *how invaluable that gift is* and not try to do something we are less suited for, like trying to be semiprofessional neuroscientists and using terms that no parent understands.

It is true that to appreciate the nuances of SPD, familiarizing ourselves with the sensory systems and having a basic, general understanding of what happens in the brain during sensory processing facilitates treatment planning for children with SPD. We can hear all you parents thinking, *"But wait! Hold on a minute! That sounds so difficult! I don't want to know all about the brain! I just want to know what to do to help my child!"* Don't worry—we know. So before we get into more details about the brain, let's talk about how much we as parents and caretakers *need to know* about the specific functioning of the brain to be able to help our "sensational" children.

Most of us don't have degrees in neuroscience, neurophysiology, or neuroanatomy. Do we ever *look* at the brain? No. We look at *behavior*. Parents are in charge of loving their children, and they look at their child's gifts and come to us because of concerns they have about their child's challenges. Teachers are responsible for fostering our children's academic progress, and they come to us when they think we can help a child improve in specific school-related skills. Therapists are not in the "center circle" of the child, family, and friends. Therapists evaluate sensorimotor functioning, as well as social participation, self-control, self-esteem, and many other aspects of the individual. Therapists implement programs that improve the quality of life for all family members.

We believe that a general working knowledge of the brain is enough for most of us. Therefore, this book presents a brief overview of the sensory systems and suggests what is *suspected* neurologically in some of the subtypes of SPD. Our explanations of the underlying neurological pieces are simplified. Instead of hypothesizing about neurological attributions, we focus on activity modifications for specific sensory subtypes. We are deliberately very careful with neurological language throughout the book, and we recommend that you be cautious about it, too. We try to focus on what *we really do know,* which is rooted in observable behavior.

So, we'll make a deal with you. We will present a brief overview of the sensory systems and describe *suspected* neurological issues noted in various subtypes of SPD, *only when evidence exists to support our beliefs.* These will be simple statements that are not intended to tell the entire neurophysiologic story.

Just so you know, there was a happy ending to the Janssen's story. Four weeks later, I saw the family when they were leaving the STAR Center. Cyril was all smiles as he said, "We want to thank you so much! You have given us our boy back. Now we feel like real parents again, and we know what we should do versus what our therapist back home should handle. And thanks for making time to have your occupational therapist video-chat with our therapist at home. That's been great, too. Look at Anthony now! He's teasing his mother! We play games all the time. We laugh, and we have stopped trying to be Anthony's therapist and have returned to being his mom and dad. We are a family again!"

What Is SPD?

Sensory Processing Disorder, in simple terms, is difficulty taking in and interpreting sensory information so that an appropriate response can be generated. We believe there are six subtypes of SPD, which will be summarized in the following chapter. But before we get into the subtypes, let's look briefly at our eight sensory systems, so we can understand their role in SPD.

The Eight Sensory Systems

Our eight sensory systems receive and send important information to the brain from both inside and outside our bodies. Each sensation may have a slightly different meaning to each person, depending on how an individual's brain interprets sensory input. On the basis of personal differences, such as varying interpretations of sensory information or the associations we have with sensory experiences, the brain generates a response (such as a motor or behavioral response) that is unique to the individual. So, to be able to design and implement helpful treatment activities for kids with sensory challenges, it is important on a behavioral level to have some understanding about how sensory input either supports or challenges each child.

The eight sensory systems include the five basics we all learned in school: sound, sight, smell, taste, and touch. In addition, two other critical sensory systems have come to be consistently included in the SPD and sensory-integration literature because they are crucial to treatment:

- Vestibular system: Movement of the head in relation to gravity

- Proprioception: Pressure in the muscles and joints

Finally, there is one more *very basic* internal sensory system, called "interoception."[5] Interoceptors are internal sensors that provide a sense of what our internal organs are feeling. Hunger and thirst are examples of interoception.

Let's tackle each sensory system, one by one.

Auditory system.—The auditory system processes and interprets information that is heard. Auditory processing includes the ability to detect sound located near the right versus the left ear and separate sounds heard in one ear from the other ear. Auditory processing also allows us to discern a specific auditory target, such as a teacher's voice, from background noise, such as general noise in the classroom. One part of the auditory system, the cochlea, is closely associated with the vestibular system, and, thus, the use of vestibular and auditory stimulation can be quite beneficial in improving language.

Processing problems in the auditory system can wreak havoc, especially in school. Although a child's hearing may not be affected, the sounds he hears, such as words, are often missing specific pitches, which make it sound as if the person talking has marbles in her mouth. Another difficulty is *hyperacusis,* where a child's hearing is too sensitive. When a noisy fire engine goes by, it is common for a child with hyperacusis to feel extreme disruption, cover his ears, and cry. It can take hours to calm him down fully. Yet another variation is a child who cannot discriminate similar sounds. Asking this child to "get your book" may be interpreted as "let us look," and so on. Children with this auditory-processing issue are in serious trouble when it comes to following directions and are often mislabeled as "slow" learners.

Visual system.—The visual system involves the eyes bringing in information about the surrounding environment. Our visual system is the most important way we determine where we are in space. The other systems that work with the visual system in this function are primarily the vestibular, proprioceptive, and tactile systems. Together, these systems allow us to make sense of the world around us, to move about in response to that world, to perform motor actions related to what is seen (such as catching a ball), and to understand the body language of others. To process more abstract visual-processing information, such as reading, writing, spelling, or calculation, abilities in the lower-level, basic areas of the visual system must be functioning well.

Children with visual-processing difficulties often have significant difficulties at school. At the far end of the visual processing–disorder spectrum are those who can't read. But the more subtle difficulties, where children think a square and a rectangle look the same, or a *b* and a *d* are identical, can be extremely frustrating and can result in children feeling they are "dumb" or "stupid." Other aspects of visual processing difficulties, such as picking out a figure from a complex and busy background, can lead to problematic behaviors. For example, when the child goes through the cafeteria line, he or she picks up a fork instead of a spoon from the silverware slots; or when selecting one of each shape to make a jack-o-lantern in art class, the child does not end up with the correct shapes (she might select three squares instead of a triangle and two squares).

Olfactory system.—The olfactory system is one of the first sensory systems to develop. Information from things you smell can quickly affect emotions and call up memories of emotional events. Smell is important not only for enjoying what you eat and being aware of danger (such as detecting something burning), but also to *be able* to eat. Many children have such severe sensitivities that they cannot have dinner with their families, go with their friends into stores that have a "funny" smell, or eat in restaurants.

Gustatory system.—The system that provides information regarding the *quality* of foods and liquids we taste is the gustatory sense, sometimes called the "gustation" sense. While this sense may not seem very important, many children with severe feeding problems have disrupted gustatory systems. Some disruptions are so severe that the only way a child can be fed and grow is by having a gastrostomy tube ("g tube") inserted into her stomach. The social and self-esteem sequelae of this fairly intense procedure can have long-term consequences. For some of these children, addressing sensory problems can significantly benefit their overall feeding therapy.

Tactile system.—The tactile system processes sensory information gathered from the skin. This is our largest sensory system and plays an important role in behavior. Touch sensations are some of the earliest sensations an infant feels. Different types of sensory receptors in the skin receive information about touch, pressure, texture, heat, cold, and pain.

When it comes to the treatment of SPD, one important attribute of the touch system is that we have *two* subsystems for touch perception. The first is the *protective system*, which makes us respond quickly to any stimulus that is perceived as being potentially harmful. Often, this unexpected stimulus takes the form of light touch. For example, the protective touch system feels the little spider crawling up your arm that you respond to by slapping quickly, without thinking.

The second touch subsystem is our *discriminative system*. This system gathers detailed information about characteristics of things that are external to our inner environment—things that we feel. This system tells us the difference between hard and soft, smooth and rough, hot and cold.

Both systems must work well together for our behavior to be "normal." Often in SPD, we see an overactive protective system (sometimes called *tactile defensiveness*). Another symptom we see in SPD is the inability to know what is felt. For example, a child has trouble feeling the buttons on her coat; therefore, she has trouble buttoning it. The latter problem involves difficulty with the discriminative touch system, also known as *poor tactile discrimination*.

Many children who are referred for therapy have problems with their tactile systems. A child can be either too sensitive, pulling away from every meaningful contact (starting with cuddling as an infant), or not sensitive enough (basically uninterested in communicating through touch). Both of these tactile problems can set up cycles of misunderstanding between a child and his caretaker. This can result in an inability to relate socially that can continue into adulthood.

Vestibular system.—The vestibular system responds to sensations about the position of your head in relation to gravity, such as, "*I'm moving up,*" or "*I'm moving down.*" It also responds to sensations of your head accelerating or decelerating, as in, "*I'm moving faster*" and "*I'm moving slower.*"

In SPD, we see five types of vestibular difficulties. The first type is called *gravitational insecurity,* where a person is uncomfortable with changes in movement. This can manifest as a *fear of movement* (such as climbing, jumping, leaning back, and riding in a car) and/or falling. The second type is an *overresponsivity* to movement, where a person feels nauseous, dizzy, or bad during or after movement in space, such as after spinning on a merry-go-round. The third difficulty is accurately feeling one's position in space. This type of problem may be called a *discriminative problem,* similar to what we discussed earlier with the tactile system. I overheard this interchange recently: "James, you're sliding off the big ball," said Miss Nikki. "I know, Miss Nikki, but I can't tell which way."

Fourth, some children may not feel movement in any direction, and these children are often called *underresponsive* to movement input. When moved in space, such as lying in a hammock that is swinging back and forth vigorously, they appear bland and unaware of the input. When Dad throws them into the air and catches them, they do not laugh and giggle and indicate they want more.

The fifth type is only a problem if it causes behavioral or motor difficulties. This problem manifests as wanting more than the usual amount of movement. This is the child who runs around incessantly, fidgets and moves without end, and wants more and more and more when swinging, spinning, or jumping. At the STAR Center, we have learned a profound lesson—there are children who want what we call *fun fast*. These movers and shakers just love to move and get great joy from the experience. We distinguish these children from those who want *too fast* (which we also call *too much fast*). We believe that this is an important distinction to make, because some children seem to be almost *addicted* to movement and go "way past" *fun fast*. This last group we call *sensory cravers,* to distinguish them from children who just love to move. When *sensory cravers* move, they do not become joyous—they disintegrate, become disorganized, and often scream or throw a tantrum if they cannot have more.

The vestibular system has many facets that obviously affect function. One of the least-appreciated connections is the association between the vestibular and hearing systems, which are connected anatomically. Often we find, for example, that a specific type of vestibular stimulation combined with auditory input results in an improved ability to communicate.

The effects of vestibular dysfunction may seem abstract, but they are actually quite profound. Your relationship to the earth is defined by gravity, which helps you sense where you are in space. If you are unaware of the vestibular stimulation you are receiving or if you are overly sensitive to this stimulus, your ability to play with other children may be severely impacted. Play, especially in the early years, involves moving your head around in space. Whether you are rolling down a hill, swimming and goofing off, or riding your bike, if your vestibular sensory system is not functioning well, you will have difficulties, and those problems will set you apart from your peers.

Proprioceptive system.—This sensory system allows us to feel changes in the length of our muscles and the position of our joints. The proprioceptive system sends us sensory information caused by stretching and contracting our muscles and by bending, straightening, pulling, and compressing our joints. Because there are so many muscles and joints in the body, the proprioceptive system is extremely large.

Our proprioceptors give us information about the position of our body parts. Most proprioception is done unconsciously, without thinking about it. We don't have to look at our arms and legs to know where they are and exactly what position they are in. For example, once you've learned how to ride a bike, you don't have to watch your feet pedaling to make the bicycle wheel go around.

Like the tactile and vestibular sensory systems, the proprioceptive system plays a large role in sensory-based treatment. Many children have difficulty judging how hard they are pushing another child and get into trouble without meaning to. Children with poor proprioception are the ones who erase right through their paper because they push so hard. Most importantly, if you can't feel your muscles and joints well, you have no sense of where your body is in relation to people or objects around you. Without a precise definition of where your body parts are located in relation to your surroundings, you can't play sports, write legibly, or button your jacket. Proprioception is the foundation for many activities that involve other sensory systems.

Interoceptive system.—Last but not least, we have interoception. What a big word for a pretty simple idea! Interoception provides sensations from our internal sensors near our organs, such as our stomach, intestines, and bladder. This system provides information about how our bodies feel inside. For example, interoceptors tell us when we are hungry or thirsty and what's going on inside our bladder and bowels.

A child who is always in the nurse's office with a headache, a tummy ache, a pain in her side, or a problem with another body organ will get a reputation at school as being a baby or a wimp or being sickly. And then perhaps that child starts to think of herself that way, too. It's a downward cycle of failure that is hard to stop. Interoception is the ability to feel the sensations from your internal organs, which is likely key in learning to control your bladder and bowels. Toilet-training problems become critical issues for boys and girls, especially as they graduate from preschool.

So these are the eight sensory systems in a nutshell. The little snippets of difficulties noted previously are just that—"little peeks." They are meant not to be complete descriptions, but just enough to whet your appetite for what you'll be reading in the remaining chapters in this book—one on each subtype of SPD.

At this point, you may be tempted to skip to the chapter you think describes your child's subtype. Of course, not only freedom of speech, but also freedom of reading is a founding principle of our country! However, we encourage you to read this book in the order in which it is written. Why? Because almost all children with SPD have multiple senses that are affected, and many have more than one subtype of SPD. One child may have two senses that are overresponsive, and the same child may have three other senses that are underresponsive. For example, a common combination is a child who is overresponsive to touch and sound but who craves movement and proprioception. Reading straight through the book will provide you with a more complete understanding of SPD than if you focus on one specific subtype.

SPD Defined

Each of us has unique neurological wiring. Some of us process input with more efficiency, and others with less efficiency. This accounts in part for our "individual differences"—what makes us distinct from each other. What makes us functional is whether or not we can make sense out of the environment and respond to both internal signals and external demands with meaningful and purposeful actions. "Typically developing" children have efficient wiring systems and are able to enjoy childhood and experience fun, with many moments of excitement and pleasure. They can make and keep friends, have satisfying experiences with their families, interact well at school, and appreciate the beauty of nature and the wonder of the world around them.

During the school years, typically developing children may engage in many extracurricular activities and have hobbies and interests that help define them as individuals. They may look forward to going to school for the most part, where learning is undertaken and skills acquired. Their skills help them to participate in fine- and gross-motor activities and to form the basis for effective speech and communication. Many functions of the sensorimotor systems become automatic, freeing up the higher brain functions for thinking, planning, and dreaming. Active involvement at home, at school, and in social settings helps these children develop a solid foundation to create a meaningful future.

Critical to this successful negotiation of one's life path is the ability to process sensory input automatically. Sensory processing requires a complex set of brain functions, including detecting, modulating, integrating, and accurately interpreting information received through the sensory systems. Processing sensory input enables meaningful responses to be made in the motor, language, cognitive, behavioral, and other related domains. Sensations inform people about the characteristics of their internal feelings and the qualities of their external surroundings. Our recent research suggests three primary classifications of SPD and a total of six separate subtypes. What defines a subtype of SPD is a controversial subject in the field. That's because no one has enough data to really answer the question of exactly *what the SPD subtypes are,* so most models are theoretical in nature. When the empirical data are lacking, people argue on the basis of belief systems rather than knowledge.

The newest classification scheme was suggested first by Miller, Lane, Cermak, Anzalone, and Koomar;[6] later refined by Miller, Lane, Cermak, Anzalone, and Osten;[7] and further clarified by Miller in 2006.[8] This classification scheme (also called *nosology*) is based on our best educated guess from our existing data of what patterns or subtypes of SPD exist. Our related empirical evidence is only now beginning to appear in the research literature.[9] The patterns are expected to shift over the years, as more scientific evidence becomes available. In fact, in the absence of hard, objective data, such as genetic evidence, a continuously shifting model makes sense as new data are published to support or refute the existing model. Over time and as our knowledge grows, we come closer to the actual subtypes. We may ultimately find that SPD is not a unitary disorder, but actually two or three separate disorders that should not be grouped together under one umbrella term.

Some clinicians find this situation distressing. They want to "know" what the subtypes are, and they don't want the patterns to keep evolving and changing. But for a researcher, change is important and positive. It suggests that you have additional clarifying data that bring you closer to the "truth." We use quotes because in the field of neurodevelopmental and behavioral disorders, "truth" is only *approached* but not *reached*—at least not until a more objective method of diagnosis is developed by the scientific community.

So, what does this mean for parents? Not much! Parents need to have evaluations conducted by clinicians who have been well trained in SPD and have studied with and been mentored by experienced, high-level experts in the field. For parents and children, what matters are the strengths and challenges of the individual child. We believe that the more elements of SPD that can be tested and observed individually, the better understanding a clinician will have of any particular child. If these elements can be addressed separately, then the child can be "put back together" within the context of his or her family. So, we propose using the newest nosology to evaluate all the elements that might be affecting a particular child. Then, all the pieces of knowledge gained can be put back together to paint a picture of the whole child.

Subtypes of SPD

SPD occurs on a spectrum, with mildly affected individuals coping with their sensory challenges to more severely affected individuals, who have great difficulties with performing routine daily tasks. The latter group has difficulty functioning scholastically, vocationally, recreationally, and in social settings. These children have motor problems and quite often exhibit pronounced anxiety, withdrawal, depression, behavioral problems, alcohol and/or substance abuse (depending on their age), or combinations of these problems.

SPD has been shown in research to affect 5% to 16% of children.[10,11] The causes of SPD have not yet been identified in definitive research, but a few studies implicate genetic factors,[12] birth complications,[13] and environmental factors[14] as potential causes.

Here is a summary of the six basic subtypes of SPD. The current, most evolved figure denoting how we now perceive the nosology in SPD is shown in **Figure 1.1**.

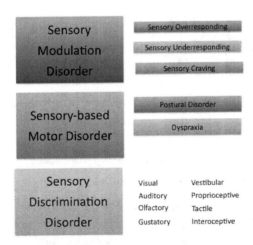

Figure 1.1. The six SPD subtypes. Note: Thank you to Dr Sarah A. Schoen for her assistance in editing these definitions.

An overview of each subtype follows. Along the way, you will "meet" children who demonstrate salient behaviors and characteristics specific to each one.

Sensory Modulation Disorder

Sensory modulation disorder has three subtypes: sensory overresponsivity, sensory underresponsivity, and sensory craving. These subtypes are described in detail in chapters 4-6.

Sensory overresponsivity.—Toby is a child with sensory overresponsivity. He appears quite skeptical of who you are and wonders what you might do to him or what you might try to make him do. You may feel as if there is a barrier of barbed wire around Toby, and it's hard to get close to him. It feels like Toby is protecting himself from everyone and everything. It takes time to get to know who Toby is, but once his guard comes down, there is an intensity to Toby that no other child may possess. The process of getting to know Toby is like unpeeling an artichoke to get at the meaty insides.

Children with sensory overresponsivity are very reactive to small amounts of external and internal stimuli. They often experience a sense of overload because they are easily aroused by stimulation in one or multiple sensory systems. Sensory information for children like Toby is experienced as painful and scary, triggering a flight-or-fight reaction in which the child wants to run away and hide.

Sensory underresponsivity.—Sergio is having a snack with his classmates in Ms Garcia's classroom. The room is noisy, with kids laughing and talking. Sergio, a first-grade student, is having pudding for a snack. He has sensory underresponsivity. When you look at him, the first image that comes to mind is a tiny weeping willow tree, melting and seeping toward the ground. What's most intriguing is that in spite of all the noise around the class, Sergio seems impervious to it and remains in a dreamy, lethargic-looking state. You call to him, "Sergio," but there's no response. You try again, a little louder this time, but still no response. Hmm. This time you try coming closer, and with a little shoulder tap and louder voice, you repeat, "Sergio!" "Oh hi," Sergio says, noticing you in the classroom for the first time. "I'm Miss Nikki," you say. "Do you want to play a game?" Sergio responds with a blank stare, and then after a pause shakes his head "No!"

Children with sensory underresponsivity process sensory information from internal and external environments slowly, requiring increased frequency and/or intensity before they notice sensory input. Children like Sergio appear to have a poor inner drive and a lack of initial desire to explore and play.

Sensory craving.—Rebecca is an overzealous little kindergartener. She rushes over to greet you and says, "I like your red hair and your shiny necklace! Hey, what's all that stuff you're carrying around?" She moves closer to you with no awareness of personal boundaries and is now practically sitting on your lap, anxious to see your new toys and games. She starts to pull some of the toys out of your arms.

"Wait one minute," you say to her. Rebecca moves quickly, and her actions are somewhat unpredictable.

You say, "Hey Rebecca, what did one penny say to the other?"

"I don't know, what?" answers Rebecca.

"Let's get together and make some sense!"

She smiles and retorts, "Do you know where a snowman keeps his money?"

"No" you reply, "Where?"

"In a snow bank!" she says, laughing.

Rebecca has a witty sense of humor that makes you both smile. You connect emotionally for a brief moment, each of you acknowledging that you are having fun and kidding around. Okay, so for the moment you have Rebecca's undivided attention. You turn around to get something from your bag that you brought for Rebecca to play with, and when you turn back to her, she is gone. The 5 seconds you dug around in your bag was too long for her to wait—she lost interest and is now off doing something else in another location.

Sensory craving is a subtype that is different than both sensory overresponsivity and underresponsivity. A prevalent belief in the field is that sensory craving (or *sensory seeking,* as it is commonly called) is caused by children not getting enough stimulation. Those who believe this generally think that sensory cravers, like sensory underresponders, need strong intensity and frequent and large amounts of stimulation to "fill them up."

We have found this to be somewhat of a myth. We have data that suggest that children who crave sensation, like Rebecca, are in their own modulation category, which is different from children with sensory over- and underresponsivity.

Unlike children with sensory over- and underresponsivity, sensory cravers become more disorganized with sensory input, unless it's provided in a very specific manner, with a functional goal and for a specific parameter of time. More details on sensory craving are described in chapter 6.

Sensory-based Motor Disorder

Two subtypes of SPD fall under this category—postural disorder and dyspraxia.

Postural disorder.—It is circle time in Ms Tello's room, and Elena and her classmates are all sitting on the carpet. Elena stands out among her peers, with her body slumped over so close to the floor that her little trunk is in a "C" shape. Elena seems genuinely uncomfortable while trying to sit up. She looks even more uncomfortable when she attempts to move. The class stands up, and Elena's knees buckle beneath her. Her peers take a break and are going outside to the playground. Elena reaches out to grab your hand for assistance in getting up. "Can we play here instead? I don't really like going on the playground. I'm not a good climber. I hate the swings," she says, winded and speaking in short sentences.

Children with postural disorder have difficulty processing sensory stimulation from the proprioceptive (information from the joints and muscles of the body) and vestibular (sense of movement in relation to the pull of gravity) systems. Like Elena, they feel uncomfortable with body-position changes. They have weak muscle tone and difficulty sustaining a stable body position while moving. As infants, they may cry or whimper when being moved around by their caretakers. Details for helping children with postural disorder are provided in chapter 8.

Dyspraxia.—Arturo is tripping over his own untied shoelaces and falling down onto the floor. "Oh boy," you think. The teacher begins a morning exercise routine, and Arturo stands back, watching the other kids do the routine. This routine was taught by his teacher yesterday, and the class has quickly caught on, with the exception of Arturo.

"Arturo, can you show me how these steps are done so I can do the exercises too?" you ask.

Arturo answers, "Just watch, you will see how my friends do it."

"Okay," you think, "He might know what needs to be done, but he just can't seem to organize the steps to do it."

Arturo and other children with dyspraxia have difficulty making a plan for action. They often prefer to watch others, because they are challenged by unfamiliar movements that have multiple steps, like the new exercises shown to the class. Dyspraxia is further described in chapter 9.

Sensory discrimination disorder.—Having talked to Ramira's teacher the day before, when you get to her classroom, you have brought extra supplies of paper, crayons, and pencils. You watch Ramira color a flat sheet that is then supposed to be cut with scissors and taped together to make a box **(Figure 1.2)**.

Ramira is using so much force that the crayons keep breaking, and she is making holes in the sheet. She grasps the scissors upside-down to make cuts, and her cutting strokes are small and way outside the lines. When she tries to tape the sides of the box together, she has trouble manipulating the tape, and it

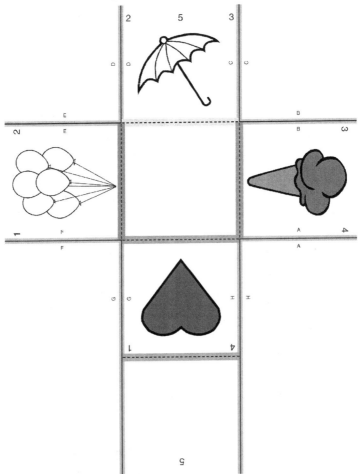

Figure 1.2. A typical school art project: making a paper box. *Source:* The Goal-Oriented Assessment of Life Skills Test, Research Edition, by Miller, Oakland, and Herzberg (Western Psychological Services, 2011).

gets all tangled up in her fingers. Ramira clearly has no idea which sides of the box are taped to each other. She is becoming extremely frustrated.

"Hi Ramira. Your teacher asked me to come see you today to find out if I could help you with projects like this."

In a loud voice Ramira responds, "I don't need help! I'm done now anyway."

Ramira stands up and pushes her chair under the table. The desk moves 2 feet forward because she uses so much force. Ramira seems unaware that the desk moved unnecessarily.

Sensory discrimination disorder is the third major pattern of SPD. Children with this subtype have difficulties interpreting and distinguishing messages within one or more sensory systems, which can result in confusion, frustration, and often very slow work. In the preceding vignette, Ramira demonstrated discriminatory challenges with the following systems: visual (difficulty seeing where to cut), proprioceptive (coloring through the paper), and auditory (using a voice level inappropriate for the setting). Children with sensory discrimination disorder have subtle problems, which are often more cognitive than motor in nature. Sensory discrimination disorder is described in detail in chapter 7.

Lori Ann's Story

Lori Ann is a 9-year-old girl with SPD. Although she gets good grades in school, she has a hard time making new friends and prefers to be alone at lunch and at recess. She cries at the drop of a hat, and she's called a "weirdo" by the more "popular" girls. She tells the other children to leave her alone and avoids physical contact with peers and adults at school. She bundles up with sweaters and coats, regardless of the season and ambient temperature, and she never stays after school to participate in extracurricular activities. She often complains of headaches and stomachaches and spends a great deal of time in the school nurse's office. She continues to have "bathroom accidents" during the school day and often has to go to the nurse's office to change into a new set of clothes. Her parents have taken her to an endless list of doctors and specialists to rule out medical and physical issues with regard to her somatic issues and complaints. Nothing medical has been discovered as a cause for Lori Ann's toilet problems, stomachaches and headaches, issues in regulating body temperature, and high anxiety.

Lori Ann talks to her therapist and confides that she gets really scared when going to special classes, lunch, and recess. She says she hates to ride the bus home from school. She is not able to explain why these transitions are so bothersome and anxiety provoking. Her therapist understands that the anxiety is not necessarily related to "not being able to transition." Instead, it stems from the difficulty and discomfort Lori Ann experiences when she has to organize sensations in loaded, unpredictable environments. Some environments that are familiar and more predictable (like her home and classroom) are more comforting for Lori Ann, who has sensory overresponsivity and sensory discrimination disorder. The more sensation that is present in the environment (such as in "special" classes like music, gym, art, recess, and the bus), the more anxiety Lori Ann feels. Lori Ann is one of many children with SPD.

In the following chapters, you will meet other children who, like Lori Ann, have sensorimotor issues. These issues result in a child experiencing multiple challenges—emotionally, physically, psychologically, and socially. Our suggested strategies and problem-solving methods are designed to help these children experience success.

Revealing *"A SECRET"* to Intervention

Individual Differences

What makes SPD so confusing when trying to obtain an accurate diagnosis is that there are eight sensory systems and six SPD subtypes, and an individual child can exhibit competencies and/or challenges in one or more of the eight sensory systems. He or she can also have one or more subtypes. So you do the math! With eight senses and six subtypes, that means there are 8 factorial x 6 factorial, or *29,030,400 different possible combinations* of types or variations of sensory challenges. (We conducted a permutation with seven options instead of six, as one additional subtype category is "normal" when considering diagnosis. Many thanks to Abby Eurich at Yale and Elliott Hedman at the Massachusetts Institute of Technology for assistance with calculating this amazing number of variations in SPD phenotypes!)

A child could have many combinations of subtypes, involving many sensory systems. For example, he or she could display sensory overresponsivity in the auditory and tactile systems, but be sensory craving in the vestibular and proprioceptive systems. If that were true, his profile would look like that noted in **Table 2.1.**

Since you can have one, two, or any combination of subtypes up to six, and one, two, or any combination of sensory systems up to eight affected, no wonder children with SPD do not all resemble each other.

Each patient we treat manifests different symptoms. A child could be underresponsive visually but overresponsive to auditory stimuli. More simply put, a kid who seems impervious to the spectacle of a county fair—the whirl of the roller coaster, the mirrors of the funhouse, the bright lights of the Ferris wheel—may be driven to distraction by a pencil tapping on the other side of the classroom. All the variations in symptoms make SPD incredibly confusing to diagnose.

Table 2.1. Understanding the Wide Variety of SPD Variations—A Sample Profile of a Child with SPD

SPD Subtype	Visual System	Auditory System	Gustatory System	Olfactory System	Tactile System	Vestibular System	Proprioceptive System	Interoceptive System
Sensory Overresponsivity		X						
Sensory Underresponsivity					X			
Sensory Craving						X	X	
Postural Disorder								
Dyspraxia								
Sensory Discrimination Disorder								

Families often come to the STAR Center with one big request—"Please give my child a sensory diet"—with static lists of exercises and perhaps "dos and don'ts" for their kids. But, given the seemingly endless ways SPD can affect children, such a one-dimensional approach cannot begin to address the diverse needs of the children we see.

STAR Center clinicians, as well as therapists we have trained in our mentorship program, help parents understand their child's specific sensory challenges, learn ways to reframe behavior, and rediscover how to have fun as a family. Being trained to solve problems based on what is happening *in context* means that you don't have a static list of activities stuffed into your purse or under a pile on your kitchen counter. Instead, you use the *principles* you've been taught to ask questions about what strategies might help your child move forward. We call that strategy "A SECRET," and parents who learn how to work this problem-solving process into their lives notice huge changes in their kids' attitudes and overall improvement in their family's quality of life. As the adage says, we find that teaching families—including a child with SPD—to "fish" goes much further than giving them a fish each time they need one.

Maria's Story

Maria is a 3-year-old girl from Romania, who was adopted after spending more than 2 years in an orphanage with minimal environmental stimulation or emotional interaction. In Romania, she slept in a small crib in a dimly lit room with 20 other babies. She was rarely allowed to crawl or move anywhere except inside her tiny crib. When she was fed, her bottle was propped against a blanket, and she was rarely held or cuddled. When she was old enough to hold the bottle herself, her caretakers paid no attention to her at all.

Melinda and Denzel Walton had been looking forward to this adoption for over a year, dreaming about the beautiful baby girl they knew only from a photograph. They despaired when they finally went to Romania to pick Maria up a few months after her 2nd birthday. She alternated constantly between fits of screaming and staring blankly into space.

When we saw Maria at the STAR Center, she had turned 3 years old and had been with the Walton family for several months. **Table 2.2** summarizes her sensory modulation by each sensory system observed during her occupational-therapy evaluation.

Table 2.2. Maria's Sensory Modulation Functioning in Each Sensory System

Sensory System	Sensory Modulation Subtype		
	Sensory Overresponsivity	Sensory Underresponsivity	Sensory Craving
Visual	X		
Auditory		X	
Tactile	X		
Smell		X	
Taste		X	
Proprioception			X
Vestibular			X
Interoception	X		

It was clear that Maria demonstrated overresponsivity in her visual and tactile systems. Her visual sensitivity was understandable, given that her body hadn't adjusted to sunlight. Naturally, she was sensitive to touch (also called *tactile defensiveness*) because she had hardly been touched, other than when her diaper needed changing or when she was being poked and prodded during checkups and vaccinations.

Notice the underresponsiveness in Maria's auditory system. When the Waltons called her name across the room, she wouldn't turn to look at them. In the orphanage, she was rarely spoken to, and her brain had no opportunity to learn to process sound. She was able to hear just fine, but she seemed unable to determine the direction of sound or discriminate between similar sounds. It was all just general "noise" to her.

Likewise, Maria's olfactory (smell) and gustatory (taste) systems were also underresponsive. This was due to the orphanage's completely bland offerings of mushy food, with an occasional piece of meat stirred in. A diet with no variety of flavors or textures did nothing to stimulate Maria's arousal level to a state in which she could adequately process gustatory or olfactory sensations. She was completely disinterested in eating. Nothing seemed to entice her— not sweet cookies, salty French fries, or even colorful lollipops. (See the end of chapter 5 for further discussion of the influence of foods.)

Soon after being adopted by the Waltons, Maria learned to walk-run. The couple was thrilled. They had been told she might not ever walk. But now

No Longer A SECRET

that she was upright, all she seemed to do was walk-run at full speed, with her bottom tilted upward and her knees stiff. She'd keep moving quickly, even if it meant crashing into people or furniture. When she crashed, she turned around and ran in the opposite direction. Maria never seemed to get enough movement. The Waltons gave her the freedom to keep running, even though they noticed she became more aimless and disorganized the more she ran. On her occupational-therapy evaluation, her therapist had noted that she "craved movement." Obviously, Maria had a number of significant sensory issues that were certain to affect the quality of her life and that of her parents.

Given the number of possible combinations of sensory systems and subtypes, your child may have symptoms that are entirely different than another child who receives a diagnosis of SPD. These differences are often related to a child's brain function and neurological wiring, which develop according to genetic and environmental factors. As we saw with Maria, the types of sensory input a child experiences during infancy and early childhood often play a major role in defining his or her sensory functioning later in life.

What's critical to understand is that *accurate identification drives treatment planning*. This may seem obvious, but far too often we see evaluations of children that woefully lack in specificity. A parent may fill out a generalized, checklist-type inventory, but the therapist has not conducted an evaluation of the eight sensory systems and the six SPD subtypes. How can you even begin treatment if you don't know which systems are sensory overresponsive, sensory underresponsive, or sensory craving?

Every hour of every day brings challenges for children with SPD and their families. Neither we nor the *sensational* children we know have time to waste messing around with one-size-fits-all treatments.

Intervention: Learning A SECRET

At every break during the workshops we teach, parents and therapists come up to ask us the same question: "What should I do when [Johnny] displays [X] behavior?" Only half-jokingly, it has occurred to us to prohibit any question that starts with the words "I have a kid who..." As silly as that may sound, the only advice we can give without seeing the child is usually, "It depends." That's because every child, every family, and everyone involved in trying to help each child is different. Given all these variables—which cannot be understood without undergoing a complete evaluation—how could we possibly offer a useful answer about a child we've never seen? The point is that there isn't one silver-bullet solution for SPD. A more constructive question to ask at break time during workshops would be, "What characteristics should I be looking for in a center to get a complete evaluation that will guide me in helping my child?"

One way to approach the complex issues of treatment is to have a logical, systematic framework within which to choose the best strategy to try. The overview of such a framework was presented in *Sensational Kids: Hope and Help for Children with Sensory Processing Disorder*.[15] That approach—for which we use the acronym "A SECRET"—is designed to demystify what an occupational therapist takes into account when assessing a child's behaviors and strategizing about the next steps to take to meet his or her specific needs. Once understood, the elements of "A SECRET" give families, teachers, and therapists a framework from which to develop a plan of intervention.

A "myths and magic" atmosphere often surrounds the treatment of children with SPD and other sensory issues. We hope to demystify the process with this book. After all, once you understand "A SECRET," it's not a secret anymore! We hope that you will have a much clearer understanding of the important goals of treatment and feel that no matter what role you play in the life of a child with SPD, you're empowered to take the next step forward.

Clinical Reasoning and Problem-Solving

No two therapy sessions look alike. Therapy is individualized to the child *in context* and *in the moment*. In occupational therapy, the process of clinical reasoning is internal (for example, in the therapist's head). Because we've found that there is no substitute for parental education, at the STAR Center we conduct about 20% of our sessions for parents only (with no children present). We use that time to help families learn about the process of asking questions and searching for strategies by sampling a wide set of possible solutions.

Natalie and Ron Marx came to a parent education session and described the frequent stressful and embarrassing situations in which their son, Mathias, threw a fit every time they needed to shop in the grocery store or do anything else necessary for the survival of the family. Mathias ran the show, they said. It was his way or no way. The Marxes had no insights into what triggered Mathias's meltdowns.

Our occupational therapist, Jamie, talked to his parents about how the effects of sensations could accumulate throughout the day until some mild stimulus served as the straw that broke that camel's back. She also helped them problem-solve around how to determine how much sensory stimulation Mathias could tolerate. They discussed strategies to help him to function best when, say, a trip to the grocery store was unavoidable.

Jamie could have given Natalie and Ron a list of activities to try. But she didn't. Instead, her goal was to teach them how to think about what their son might need *in the moment*. Jamie suggested they try some of our active problem-solving techniques. We've found that teaching caretakers how to ask the "right" questions about strategies is far more useful than giving them a to-do list, such as a sensory diet. The Marxes realized that the calming effect Mathias gleaned from doing heavy work during therapy could be partially reproduced by having him push the heavy grocery cart. Natalie and Ron also figured out other strategies, including having Mathias match coupons to items on the grocery shelves and giving him a lollipop to suck on during the shopping trip. They also discussed the advantages of shopping early in the morning and for much shorter periods of time.

When the Marx family returned to therapy several days later, they not only reported a successful grocery-shopping trip, but they had applied the principles of what they had learned to other circumstances, as well.

From Theory to Action: A SECRET Treatment Model

The concept of "A SECRET" is not a list of prescribed activities; instead, it is a process of devising strategies that work to support your child at times when he or she is experiencing sensory challenges.

Let's say, for example, you're at a soccer game. Your child runs up to the ball and misses, runs up to the ball and misses again, then runs up and misses a third time. He looks devastated and starts stomping his feet and crying. Your heart starts to race and you begin to sweat as you say to yourself, "Oh no—not here, not now!" You hear whispers around you about your son being "klutzy." "Why is he on *our* team?" another child asks (of course that child needs some remediation too, but that's another story). "The coach should get rid of that kid," murmurs a parent. (By the way, if you don't know this yet, some "soccer parents" can be brutal in their quest to have a winning team.) Both you and your child are upset and at risk of having a total family meltdown.

If, *in the moment,* you can remember "A SECRET," maybe you can use each letter of the acronym to guide your child out of his downslide and yourself out of panicking on the sidelines. As defined in the book, *Sensational Kids,* each of the letters in "A SECRET" stands for a specific element that may lead to a strategy to help your child cope with challenging situations. These situations may range from public meltdowns like the one on the soccer field to total withdrawal into isolation at home. With SPD, there's no single challenging behavior, just as there's no single "right" strategy for every kid in every situation. What "A SECRET" teaches us is a strategy for how to problem-solve and how to come up with solutions to try, so that we can select among several options what might be the best strategy to try **(Table 2.3).**

The challenged area of "A SECRET" that you want to address can be found among the components in **Figure 2.1**.

```
A = Attention
  S = Sensation
    E = Emotional Regulation
      C = Culture, Context, or Current Conditions
      R = Relationship
      E = Environment
        T = Task
```

Figure 2.1. The Elements of the Acronym "A SECRET"

Table 2.3. A SECRET Method for Problem-Solving

Challenged Area	Elements from "A SECRET"						
	Attention	Sensation	Emotional Regulation	Culture/Context/ Current Conditions	Relationship	Environment	Task
Motor skills							

Step 1. Under "Challenged Area," select one challenge you wish to focus on and write it down. In this case, the challenged area is "motor skills."

Step 2. Use the elements of "A SECRET" to help you strategize a wide variety of ways you might help your child move forward in the challenged area.

Let's walk through the way this method works:

1. In the left column, write down the challenge(s) that you are going to consider, one at a time. For example, we've selected "motor skills" as the particular area that triggers inappropriate or immature responses.

2. Think about each element across the row for each of the letters in "A SECRET" and imagine possible strategies that might foster better outcomes for your child. Go from left to right and ask yourself how **A**ttention activities might help your child at soccer, for example. Think about how **S**ensation might provide the support your child needs to make soccer more fun. Then try to anticipate how **E**motional regulation might help prevent a meltdown during practice. And so on.

3. In each element of A SECRET, consider one or more strategies that might help your child at soccer.

4. Pick one or two strategies to try at next week's game.

5. Now take a deep breath and try to relax. You're no good to your child if you get worked up. And anyway, you have a plan!

Here are a few examples of how to approach each element of A SECRET, so you can begin to get the idea.

A = Attention

Could the problem be a lack of attention? What can I think of that might make soccer more interesting to my child and help him focus? You think, "My son Andrew is super smart. His coach has basically five plays, which several of the other players are struggling to memorize. Maybe Andrew's grasp of the plays can be used as an asset to the team. Can I urge Andrew to help his teammates by calling out the directions for the play in motion and helping to get the ball to a strong kicker?" (See **Table 2.4.**)

S = Sensation

How can some type of sensory input help Andrew succeed at soccer? You know that his motor skills are better after he receives lots of whole-body stimulation. And you remember that input to his muscles and joints calms him down. You could try having him do any one of the following exercises before the game to see if they might help him move and focus better. (See **Table 2.5.**)

Table 2.4. Example of Using Attention to Support Challenges in the Motor-Skill Area

Challenged Area	Elements from "A SECRET"						
	Attention	Sensation	Emotional Regulation	Culture/Context/Current Conditions	Relationship	Environment	Task
Motor Skills	Understands plays, calls them out to others, and sets up others to kick						

Table 2.5. Example of Using Sensation to Support Challenges in the Motor-Skill Area

Challenged Area	Elements from "A SECRET"						
	Attention	Sensation	Emotional Regulation	Culture/Context/Current Conditions	Relationship	Environment	Task
Motor Skills		Could introducing some kind of sensory input help? Maybe try sensory wrestling before the game, jumping on a trampoline, or doing heavy work					

Sensory wrestling.—Wrestling is a form of deep pressure that we call *heavy work*. Heavy work increases awareness of body position. In sensory wrestling, Andrew wrestles his mom or dad; he pushes as hard as he can while his parent barely moves, then the parent holds him down and he pushes hard to "escape." (Of course, ultimately he gathers so much strength that he escapes!) Try it for 15 minutes before his soccer game to see if it increases his body awareness and helps with his overall use of motor skills.

Jumping on a trampoline.—Sensory trampoline-jumping entails jumping while playing catch. Try doing this for 15 minutes before the soccer game to get Andrew "warmed up." He jumps up and down while you throw a ball to him, and he tries to match his jumps to the toss so he can catch the ball. It may increase his spatial awareness, and the overall vestibular stimulation should boost his arousal, hopefully improving his motor skills for the game.

Doing heavy work.—Maybe you are making a patio and need some bricks moved, or your bookshelf is too full and you need help moving books from one room to another. Anything that works the muscles and joints provides sensory input called *proprioceptive input*. This is helpful when children require help with sensory organization and feel overloaded and unable to focus on a given task.

These activities and others like them should help Andrew with body awareness, focus and concentration, and motor skills. Try these strategies one at a time and see which ones improve his soccer experience!

In the previous example, you selected the first two elements to focus on—**A**ttention and **S**ensation. By considering two of the seven elements individually, you are problem-solving. In real life, that's plenty to start with. But for practice, let's move on and demonstrate how each element of "A SECRET" can prompt you to think of strategies for Andrew to improve his soccer experience. Note that he is not necessarily improving in soccer skills, per se. What you care about is how he *perceives* his soccer experience, not whether he scores goals. So next, we move on to **E**motional regulation. What types of strategies might be useful to keep Andrew emotionally in control during soccer? (See **Table 2.6.**)

E = Emotional regulation

Although soccer is hard for Andrew, he wants to play because everyone else does. Work on preparing him emotionally by listening to CDs in the car as you drive to soccer (for example, check out *musicformotion.com*). Many libraries carry recordings such as Betty Mehling's "Magic Island," which empowers kids, Deb Weiss-Gelmi's "Sing Song Yoga" DVD, which harnesses energy into strength and flexibility, or Dr Rox's "Grain of Sand" CD, which uses songs and stories to teach stress management, self-acceptance, and a positive approach to challenges. If you send a winner out on the field, you'll probably get a winner back after the game—even if he doesn't score a point.

C = Culture, Context, or Current Conditions

How can you figure out a way to change the "culture," context, or current conditions of the soccer games so that Andrew—and his teammates—have a more positive soccer experience?

What we mean by "culture" here is the way things are usually done regarding customs, context, habits, or conditions that create a way of life that generates the atmosphere or *culture* of your family or classroom. For example, having everyone sit in the same seat for dinner helps create the culture of your family. In Andrew's case, his routine may entail riding the bus home after school, having a snack, and rushing off to his weekly soccer match. There are dozens of ways to change things on game days so Andrew's *culture* is different than usual. Maybe you could pick Andrew up from school, so he has a little extra time at home to rest. Or maybe you could make a ritual out of serving him a special, healthy snack and talking about winning and losing and what really matters in life. Help Andrew put things into perspective. Make him feel loved and successful as a person, no matter what happens on the soccer field. Talk about something fun you two will do together after soccer so that the game doesn't seem like the end of the day. These ideas only brush the surface, to give you an idea of "cultural" changes that might improve Andrew's experience in soccer.

If Andrew has a significant motor problem, such as dyspraxia or severe motor delays, the best thing might be to get him interested in a different, more individualized sport, such as swimming or gymnastics, which will let him go at his own pace and get his mind off soccer. That would certainly provide a different "culture" for him. (See **Table 2.7.**)

Table 2.6. Example of Using Emotional Regulation to Support Challenges in the Motor-Skill Area

Challenged Area	Elements from "A SECRET"						
	Attention	Sensation	Emotional Regulation	Culture/Context/Current Conditions	Relationship	Environment	Task
Motor Skills			Listen to positive, uplifting music on the way to the game.				

Table 2.7. Example of Using Culture to Support Challenges in the Motor-Skill Area

Challenged Area	Elements from "A SECRET"						
	Attention	Sensation	Emotional Regulation	Culture/Context/Current Conditions	Relationship	Environment	Task
Motor Skills				Pick Andrew up from school early to do some self-esteem boosting at home before soccer games.			

R = Relationships

The most powerful tool you have is *relationships*. You are the most constant influence in Andrew's life and can use that connection to soothe, support, and help balance his moods and emotions.

One important aspect of keeping children calm and focused is called co-regulation. Simply put, this refers to the ability to project a certain emotional tone onto a child. If, on the way to the soccer game, you're stressing over how Andrew will perform, chances are he'll pick up on your anxiety and start stressing out, too. Instead, if you stand at the sidelines and offer encouraging words—not only to Andrew, but to all the players (maybe even some on the other team), he will hear and respond to your feelings. And if he comes off the field hanging his head low and dragging his feet, you might empathize briefly but project your own positive feelings by reiterating the funny or high points of the game. Feelings are contagious. They spread through relationships. Keep yours as positive as possible around Andrew, and he might respond in kind. (See **Table 2.8.**)

E = Environment

Now think about Andrew's environment. Is there anything about the soccer field that's distracting Andrew? Or is there something you can to do tweak his experience or his surroundings to make the game more comfortable? Scan the environment to see what adaptations might be useful. Let's say Andrew is sensitive to light and is playing in the afternoon sun. Maybe sunglasses would help, or maybe the coach can move the game to a more shaded area. If he has auditory processing issues, maybe he's unable to hear his coach clearly. Try encouraging him to ask the coach to speak louder. Each situation is unique, but often an environmental change is all that's needed to ease the sensory challenge. (See **Table 2.9.**)

T = Task

Finally, let's consider Andrew's task in this case: playing soccer. Can you work with him in ways to improve his game? For example, practicing kicking in your backyard might hone his skills. Inviting an older child over to play soccer with Andrew could sweeten the deal. Or, enrolling him in a three-on-three soccer team instead of his school team could soften the competitive edge. (See **Table 2.10.**)

Table 2.8. Example of Using **Relationship** to Support Challenges in the Motor-Skill Area

Challenged Area			Elements from "A SECRET"				
	Attention	Sensation	Emotional Regulation	Culture/Context/Current Conditions	Relationship	Environment	Task
Motor Skills					Use your own positive attitude to influence how Andrew feels.		

Table 2.9. Example of Using **Environment** to Support Challenges in the Motor-Skill Area

Challenged Area			Elements from "A SECRET"				
	Attention	Sensation	Emotional Regulation	Culture/Context/Current Conditions	Relationship	Environment	Task
Motor Skills						Use markers along both sidelines so Andrew can better judge where he is on the field.	

Table 2.10. Example of Using **Task** to Support Challenges in the Motor-Skill Area

Challenged Area			Elements from "A SECRET"				
	Attention	Sensation	Emotional Regulation	Culture/Context/Current Conditions	Relationship	Environment	Task
Motor Skills							Play three-on-three soccer instead of the full team sport.

See? "A SECRET" isn't hard to learn. In terms of changing your child's life in a way that's geared toward increasing his happiness and the well-being of your family, it's totally doable.

Emotional Regulation

What Is Emotional Regulation?

This chapter describes emotional regulation (also referred to as *self-regulation*), which is "the process used to manage and cope with emotion-related...states that occur on a moment to moment basis. Many children express emotion states by exhibiting behaviors related to individual coping mechanisms."[16] Another way to think about the meaning of emotional regulation is to consider how complicated it is to control *your own* emotions. Think about the last really close call you had in a car because someone didn't watch where he or she was going. You probably had an instantaneous emotional response composed of three factors:

1. Your feelings (eg, anger or fear)

2. Your instantaneous thoughts related to the situation (eg, "This is just like last time when I was in an accident")

3. Unconscious physiological reactions to what happened (eg, your heart starts pumping faster)

We all respond to the combination of these factors. Our kids' responses include acting out, throwing temper tantrums, screaming, hitting, and exhibiting other "bad" behaviors.

Regulating your own emotional responses is critical to getting along in life. Usually when something bothers you, you can just let it go unless it's really important. You don't blurt out every little thought about it, because you've learned to control what stays inside your head versus what you say out loud.

Self-control and regulation are so important that a National Academy of Sciences report describes it as the primary cornerstone of early-childhood development, which affects all other developmental domains.[17] We also consider emotional regulation to be one of the most important foundations in functioning well with regard to all the subtypes of SPD.

This chapter uses examples and strategies that can apply to children of any subtype who demonstrate difficulties with regulating their emotions. A lack of control in this area is the most common reason children with SPD are referred to see occupational therapists. Research has shown that social skills and emotional regulation are two of the most important characteristics needed for success in school.[18] In addition, emotional regulation is an even better predictor of school readiness than Intelligence Quotient (IQ) scores from standardized testing.[19] Interestingly, attention regulation has been shown to correlate with measures of school readiness.[20] Even at the preschool age, regulation predicts later academic competence[21] and portends both verbal and quantitative SAT Test scores many years later.[22]

Emotional regulation includes our ability to modify our behavior as circumstances change. We must be able to adapt to changes in routines and transitions throughout the day and maintain a relatively balanced and calm yet alert and organized state. Each of us faces challenges every day that require us to cope. What might be appropriate at home (like a 13-year-old slamming a door when angry instead of yelling at his parents) might not be considered appropriate in another setting, such as school. The words 6-year-old Abdul uses to tell his brother to get out of his space—"Get out of here, you dumb-head. These toys belong to me and only me!"—certainly differ from what we hope Abdul would say to a teacher.

Emotional regulation abilities start to form in early infancy and grow in complexity over time. Infants depend almost entirely on caregivers to co-regulate their negative emotional responses. When an infant is upset, another person must intervene to adjust the baby's emotional state, often by adjusting his or her physiologic needs (eg, feeding, changing a diaper, or rocking the baby from side to side). By 6 to 8 months of age, infants begin to self-regulate their emotional states by using self-soothing actions, such as looking away from stimuli that upset them, finding their thumbs to suck, rocking their bodies, or crying to "call" their caretakers.

Toddlers between 1 and 2 years of age have enough attention control that they can often distract themselves from emotionally distressing stimuli by changing their attention to non-upsetting facets of the task, to caring relationships, or to other aspects of their environment. By 4 years of age, children begin to use more complex regulatory strategies. They can stop certain behaviors when they want to, as well as focus and shift their attention. Notably, by age 4, less external regulation is needed from parents and other caretakers for typically developing children. Evidence suggests that additional aspects of learning to regulate yourself continue even into adulthood.[23]

Older children begin to manage negative emotional responses by talking and negotiating solutions to difficult situations. Adults are usually much better at discussing situations that are emotionally disturbing and "working it out," although we all know people who aren't as skilled at this as we wish they would be! Often, children with SPD become "stuck" in an emotional regulation pattern typically seen in a younger age group. How often do we hear parents say, "Megan, act your age. You're eight, and you're acting younger than your brother, who is only six!"

Characteristics of Poor Emotional Regulation

Functioning in the world with poor emotional regulation is tough. This includes having difficulty with coping and demonstrating inflexibility when dealing with changes in routines, schedules, or caretakers. When change occurs, especially unpredictable change, a child with SPD may respond with anger, hostility, aggression, rigidity, anxiety, or depression. Some children withdraw, displaying "flat affect" (a failure to express feelings), with little to no engagement with others and "flattened" emotional responses. In other words, they exhibit a sort of *shutdown* appearance. One 17-year-old told me, "I remember when I was a little girl and my parents changed the mantelpiece in the living room. I cried, I kicked my arms and legs, and I finally went and hid behind the sofa and said I wouldn't come out until they put the old mantel back!"

Sammy's Story

Sammy is a 4-year old boy with severe issues in emotional regulation. One day he walked into daycare and his best friend, Aaron, came running up to him and gave him a big hug. Sammy put his arms around Aaron, hugging him back, and then he bit him on the shoulder. "What are you doing, Sammy?" cried his mother. "It wasn't me, Mommy," said Sammy. "It just came out. It was inside and came out by itself."

We suspect that some children are just barraged constantly with unexpected sensory stimulation, leading them to feel out of control all the time. They will do anything they can to keep things constant, even when it comes to the placement of furniture in a room or the paint colors on a wall.

In a state of poor emotional control, a child will have difficulty attending to stimuli from the environment, such as what the teacher is saying, which makes learning extremely challenging. He or she may become hyperactive, disorganized, and distractible. The exaggerated emotional responses are often accompanied by wide mood swings that can occur within minutes. It's common to see behavioral problems that interfere with peer interactions and relationships at home or at school. For adults with SPD characteristics, conflicts often flare up in relationships or at work.

People with poor emotional regulation often feel frightened and out of control. Because their feelings come on suddenly and are so extreme, they usually feel that their outbursts come from somewhere else—not from inside them. A sense of "doom and gloom" often sets in. Festering in negativity creates a pattern of unproductive behaviors that aggravates emotional states. As a result, people with poor emotional regulation often have low self-esteem and feel different and isolated from others.

Learning to Regulate Yourself

The goal is for a child to learn to actively identify when he or she needs to implement sensory strategies or activities if his or her emotions are starting to get out of control. When regulation is child-directed, it will have a longer-lasting, quicker, and more long-term effect than when it must be cued by a parent. However, many children need cuing from an adult to deal with stress, frustration, and transitions for a long time before they are ready to be independent. For example, Melanie accidentally bumped Jacob while they were standing in line. Although Jacob had been taught many self-regulation tools, his teacher saw him turn around as if to push Melanie back. The teacher said, "Jacob, remember our waiting game," cuing him to say three rhyming words before responding to Melanie's accidental intrusion. "Cat, hat, bat," Jacob called out, smiling. The instinct to hit Melanie subsided.

Self-regulation support strategies require adoption of a problem-solving approach rather than making a static, rule-bound attempt to regulate a child. The adult who is cuing the child must understand the underlying reasons for the strategies to be able to problem-solve on the spot, rather than refer to a list of activities that a therapist has written down—such as a sensory diet.

Joe's Story

Joe was in a self-contained first-grade classroom, and he was always getting into some type of trouble. He was a child who constantly craved new sensory input and was always on the move. He had a difficult time attending and regulating his behavior. He "lost it" particularly after lunch and recess. The difficulty he experienced when things were not structured, his defiance of limits, and his wild, purposeless running during recess got him into constant trouble with teachers and peers.

Joe's teacher, Miss Amanda, tried having Joe wear a weighted vest when he was in his most disorganized state. She was diligent in following through with this strategy every day, and for a few weeks, it seemed to be working.

One afternoon, about 4 weeks into the program of wearing the vest, the occupational therapist looked into the classroom after recess and saw Joe sitting at his desk, organized, regulated, and working diligently. He was not yet wearing the weighted vest. As Miss Amanda handed Joe his vest, he gave her a surprised look. Clearly, Miss Amanda was following through with the suggested sensory program, but she wasn't really reading Joe's behavior. *Joe was already feeling regulated* and didn't require any external modifications.

Miss Amanda's poor understanding of the purpose of the weighted vest and her adherence to wearing the vest on the basis of a rigid routine made it clear that she didn't understand the goals of occupational therapy (although she was trying to do what the occupational therapist had told her). The bottom line was that she was not recognizing Joe's needs.

Dependence on sensory diets often precludes teachers or parents from problem-solving. In addition, a static sensory diet doesn't help a child learn to control problematic behaviors. Inflexible regimes don't help kids actively choose strategies when they begin to experience a dysregulated state. Sensory diets generally call for the strategy at a certain time of day and leave no way to recognize improvement. In the previous example, when Joe's teacher handed him the weighted vest after recess, he took it and put it on, yet he looked at her with surprise. Miss Amanda should have been trained to identify Joe's calm and focused state when he came in from recess, acknowledge it, and commend Joe for it. Her goal should have been to begin to "read" Joe's emotional state and his arousal level and to cue him, so that over time he could become responsible for choosing appropriate regulating activities. Developing problem-solving skills will launch both Miss Amanda and Joe into an *active learning mode*. This will improve his coping skills, his ability to adjust to transitions, and his competence in dealing with other unpredictable events independently, without the help of his occupational therapist.

Emotional Regulation in Yourself

We all use self-regulation strategies to keep our emotions in control and to help us focus, attend, and increase our overall level of functioning. The state of being calm but on *ready alert* is called *homeostasis*. This state allows us to function effectively and efficiently in a wide range of environmental conditions.

How Doreit Regulates

On days when I lecture for 8 hours, I typically start chewing gum early in the morning. I've learned to keep the gum well hidden and controlled within my mouth as I lecture. Every few minutes, I will "sneak a chew," which provides calming, proprioceptive input throughout my jaw muscles. This sensory input helps me stay organized while I lecture, enhancing my ability to focus on my topic and on questions being asked. Although the gum loses its flavor pretty quickly, I continue to chew the gum to help me self-regulate.

The key to self-regulation is being able to identify your emotional state. A self-awareness survey is provided at the end of this chapter to help you recognize your own emotional states. Remember that to help an out-of-control child, you must enter the interaction in a regulated emotional state yourself.

Strategies for Emotional Regulation

Researchers have identified the following six effective strategies that parents can use to influence their child's emotional regulation.[24]

1. Teach yourself and your child to recognize emotional states.—Simple but targeted activities can be used for this purpose. If you describe your own feelings or go around the dinner table or classroom and have everyone relay their emotional states, this can be very helpful to children who are less aware of their own emotions. Another approach is to make educated guesses about their state and have them tell you if you are "right" or "wrong." Reinforce how important it is to learn to interpret cues in faces, body language, and the manner in which words are said.

One project you can do together is to cut out pictures from magazines or old family photos that you can talk about together. Point out how facial expressions relate to specific feelings. Have your child look at a picture of him- or herself. Maybe these photos trigger feelings of glee and happiness or sadness and fear. See if the child can show you how he or she was feeling when that photograph was taken. This type of activity can help the child recapture that emotional state and apply it to future situations.

Help the child read and identify emotional states by using yourself as a model. When you're feeling joy, anger, or frustration (not toward the child, obviously!), ask your child if he can identify how you feel. Ask him to identify *your* feelings and give him feedback. Hopefully this will help him begin to understand the continuum of emotional states. During times when children are calm, have them practice simple activities that can be used later when they are emotionally dysregulated to help them gain self-control. For example, lie down on the floor together and breathe deeply. It might help to put a small stuffed animal on your stomach to demonstrate how the stuffed animal moves up and down with your inhalations and exhalations, thus conveying a calming breathing pattern. The more practice your child has with methods like this, the easier it will be to use these strategies in a time of need.

2. Understand your own emotional regulation strategies.—We all have strategies that we use to help us deal with stress. Understanding what works for you can be a tremendous leap toward helping children with poor emotional regulation. Try to verbalize what strategies you use and see whether they may be helpful to children with emotional regulation difficulties.

3. Practice emotional regulation activities with your child.—See if you can interest your child in activities that will help him learn methods of self-regulation. For example, find a parent-child yoga or tae kwon do class. Meditation is a great activity that helps center emotions and thoughts. It's a way of helping your child focus and attend to one symbol, sound, or picture to help diffuse overwhelming feelings.

4. Use pretend play to practice emotional regulation strategies.— Draw from a scenario that your child doesn't like and reenact it "for pretend."

For example, play a game in which she makes believe she loves "yucky" foods (also make sure she knows that she doesn't have to eat it). This is a cognitive behavioral approach that helps to teach children how to remain controlled when faced with negative stimuli.[25] Both behavioral and subjective signs of negative emotions can change with this cognitive approach.

5. Explain and practice body-focused emotional regulation.—When your child is faced with something he or she doesn't like and feels that touching it is "yucky," (eg, finger-painting, touching shaving cream), ask him or her to pretend not to feel anything. The result of this "game" is called *suppression,* a type of body-focused response. Actively suppressing emotions decreases activation of the sympathetic nervous system and is good practice for children who commonly become overaroused by sensation.

6. Develop strategies to apply to poor emotional regulation.—Every teacher likely has at least one child in a classroom that demonstrates poor emotional regulation. To facilitate learning for all students in the class, children must trust their teacher and know that the environment will stay safe and fairly predictable.

One method that can reinforce a safe, predictable classroom environment is to have the class set a few rules—typically fewer than eight—during the first week of school.[26] Review the rules weekly.

If the rules are violated, use a disciplinary action that is related to the violation. For example, if a student writes on his desk, he could clean the top of all the desks. For more disruptive situations, teachers may find exchanging time-outs with other teachers to be effective, so the child can go to another room to calm down for 15 to 20 minutes.

Rewards are usually more effective than punishments. Most of us don't use rewards enough. Rewards such as having lunch with the teacher, calling the child's parents to praise specific activities, and using a token system that allows kids to buy gifts and/or rewarding activities may prevent many undesirable behaviors, even for children with poor emotional regulation.[26]

Helping children succeed in school is critical not only for individual students, but also for society as a whole. Research shows that emotional competence is absolutely related to a young child's academic competence.

Additional Strategies for Emotional Regulation

Here is a variety of cost-effective strategies you could use to help your child learn to identify, cope, and regulate his or her emotions.

Activity 3A. The Stoplight Bracelet Game

In this activity, use colored rubber bracelets to represent emotional states. The bracelets should be green, red, and yellow, like the colors on signs, traffic lights, and other universal visual cues **(Figure 3.1)**. Green bracelets represent a "green light," or positive state, such as happiness, confidence, satisfaction, and a sense that everything is okay with the world **(Figure 3.2)**. In this state, a child feels like, "I'm good. Things will work out!" Yellow bracelets represent the process of dysregulation—becoming unhappy, frustrated, or upset. Red bracelets represent feelings of anger, significant irritation, and impatience **(Figure 3.3)**.

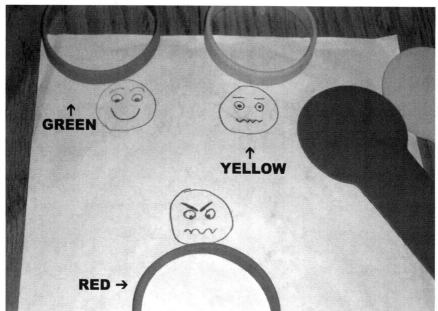

Figure 3.1. Three colored bracelets—red, yellow, and green—can be used to help children identify their emotional states.

The experience of having children wear the colored bracelets throughout the day helps them to associate their feelings with daily experiences.

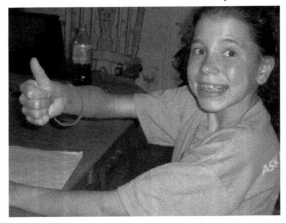

Figure 3.2. A girl demonstrates her feeling of "I'm okay" by wearing the green bracelet and signaling "Thumbs up!"

Figure 3.3. The red bracelet indicates anger or frustration.

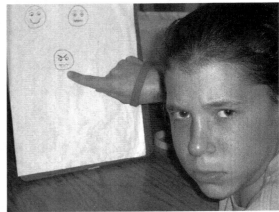

Similar to the activity used in helping children identify their emotional states by finding pictures in magazines or looking at photographs, the bracelets are worn so that words don't have to be used, and more automatic associations can be made. Talk about when the child thinks he would wear a yellow or red bracelet (and when you or another family member might wear one). Then, together, you can role-play what green, yellow, and red "feeling states" look like.

If you can help the child realize how he is feeling, you can slow down the shift from green to yellow and from yellow to red. This process will often help the child avoid red altogether. Using a cognitive technique like bracelets will help him move from an automatic "fight-or-flight" response to a "cognitively mediated" response (thinking his way through it), which provides more emotional control. We recommend that you have the child place the bracelet on his own wrist to indicate his emotional state. Mastering his own feelings will help him feel "in control." Ultimately, the child becomes empowered to appropriately choose a red, yellow, or green bracelet and develop a stronger internal awareness of emotional regulation.

Activity 3B: The Charade Game

Write all kinds of emotions on slips of paper, place them in a hat, and ask participants to select a slip and act out the emotion written on it. The other players will guess what emotion is being acted out. Another modification is to play a game in which you act out *the opposite* of what your slip of paper says. During this charade game, one boy wore a green rubber bracelet that should indicate, "I'm okay." However, his facial expression didn't correspond to the color of his bracelet, and the children in the group had to guess his emotional state and suggest the proper bracelet color **(Figure 3.4)**.

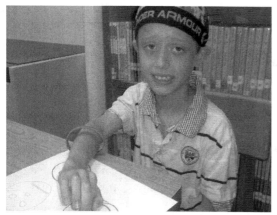

Figure 3.4. During The Charade Game, a boy wears a green bracelet but has an unhappy look on his face. The other children try to guess his emotional state and suggest the proper bracelet color.

Activity 3C: The Acting-Out-Feelings Game

Acting out different scenarios with a child helps him deal with emotional regulation externally, before having to use techniques in real situations. With repetition and practice, a child will begin to internalize a variety of self-selected regulation strategies. Children love acting and role-play, and the use of handmade puppets is a nice way of incorporating emotional expression to others **(Figure 3.5)**.

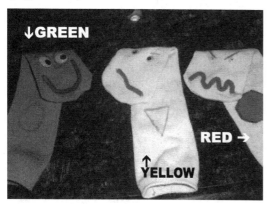

Figure 3.5. The Acting-Out-Feelings Game can be played with color-coded puppets like these, which children made out of socks.

As children practice and rehearse a variety of experiences, they become clearer about their emotional states and more in touch with their feelings in response to stimuli **(Figure 3.6)**. It's also helpful to have children practice and use self-talk to help them make sense out of their feelings. Some children may role-play for a long period of time before they really understand their own emotions.

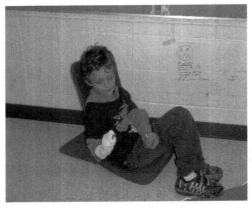

Figure 3.6. A boy uses sock puppets to rehearse different scenarios and emotional responses.

Activity 3D: Linking Activities to Emotional States

Pictures and visual cues can be useful when helping children learn to make appropriate choices of activities during emotional dysregulation (in terms of bracelets, in the "red" or "yellow" zone). As a child becomes more automatic in identifying his emotional state, you can begin to help him learn to choose appropriate activities that can be used prior to having a meltdown, throwing a tantrum, or acting out. You can present the activities to him visually, as on the cards in **Figure 3.7,** so he can choose one in an effort to self-regulate. Activities should be meaningful to the child and readily available to assist in emotional regulation.

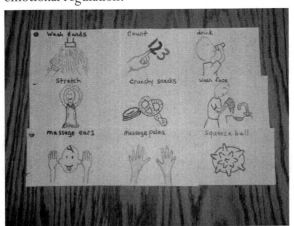

Figure 3.7. You can make cards to depict activities a child could use to help with emotional regulation. These cards were illustrated by L. Olson-Haslinger.

No Longer A SECRET

Activity 3E: The Key Ring Game

If you laminate the emotional-regulation activity cards from the previous activity, a child can place them on a key ring and then wear them on a belt or in a pocket **(Figure 3.8)**. This will cue the child to look at the cards and make active choices in balancing his emotional state.

With digital cameras, it's so easy to take photos of activities that a particular child finds organizing and useful to stay in control. Cut out and laminate the pictures, and place them on a ring for easy use.

You need to practice self-regulation with the child. This will help him become more automatic in making the connection that he can choose an alternate means of helping him balance his emotional meltdowns **(Figure 3.9)**.

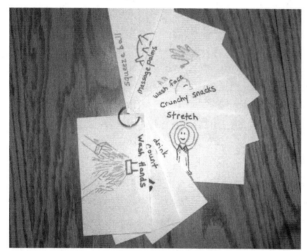

Figure 3.8. Activity cards for self-regulation can be laminated and placed on a key ring for immediate use. Cards created by K. A. Lawson.

Figure 3.9. A boy looks at his laminated self-regulation choices, which he wears around on a key ring.

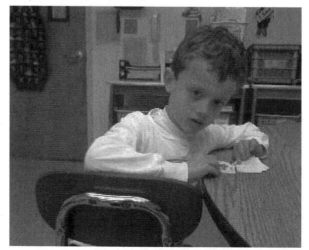

The Need for Immediate Positive Reinforcement

Most of what we've been discussing in this chapter is cognitive-behavioral strategies of one sort or another. A positive-reinforcement behavioral program is a special type of cognitive strategy in which specific, selected target behaviors (for example, getting a bottle for your little sister) are rewarded on a systematic basis. These methods are particularly effective when used consistently at both home and school. If children are actively involved in helping to design and choose elements of their own behavioral modification programs, the programs are usually more successful.

At school, having students participate with a team when they are identifying goals is often helpful. Both the child and his or her parents can assist in identifying specific behaviors that interfere with functioning at home or in natural community settings. After these problematic behaviors are selected, alternative self-regulatory behaviors can be chosen. When a child uses the alternative behavioral choice, reinforcement is provided as soon as possible after the alternative behavior is displayed. Today, with the easy access we have to gadgets such as cell phones, PalmPilots, iTouches, and the like, parents can access behavioral charts easily and provide positive reinforcement in a timely manner, even if a child is at the mall, at another family's house, or virtually anywhere. With this method, a child "earns" checkmarks, which work better if he or she can fill them in on a chart. After a certain predetermined threshold is reached, the child can earn a reward. Selecting the right reward is important—the system only works if the child has the ability to earn something he or she really wants! Most children respond best to offers of time alone with Mom or Dad on the weekend, maybe to get ice cream or a book at the library. At school, rewards such as free-play time, stickers, small toys, prizes, and other items can also be effective in reinforcing a child's selection of the target, "controlled" behavior.

Richard's Story

Richard, a second-grader, had difficulty completing classroom tasks that involved any visual-motor skills, such as cutting with scissors, writing, and coloring. He whined and protested throughout the morning whenever he was required to complete this type of activity. We found that playing on the playground equipment during recess motivated Richard. His teacher said that there were five activities that the class needed to complete in the mornings prior to lunch and recess. This became the theme for the positive-reinforcement behavioral chart we made for Richard. We made a "puzzle" of a playground slide, with five pieces. He earned one "piece" of the puzzle after he completed each of the five activities without whining **(Figure 3.10)**. When he had earned all five puzzle pieces, he completed the puzzle and earned 5 extra minutes on the playground that day. With this method, his self-regulation abilities were reinforced, and he felt better about himself because "He was the boss of his behavior."

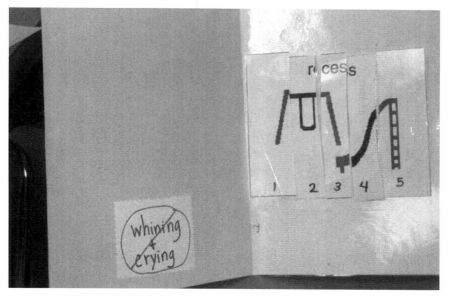

Figure 3.10. A positive-reward chart like this one can be used for reinforcements such as earning extra time on the playground. For each activity a child accomplishes without whining or crying, the child earns one piece of the "puzzle." When the puzzle is complete, the child is rewarded with extra playground time. This chart was developed by L. Carroll.

Emotional Regulation

Summary of Emotional Regulation Guidelines

Keep these three guidelines in mind when you are working with a child who has poor emotional regulation:

1. Actively involve the child in making choices and in developing his own strategies for self-regulation. He will self-regulate more by knowing how to identify his emotional states. When a child buys into the fact that the precipitating variables are contributing to his poor emotional regulation, the path to self-regulatory recovery has begun.

2. Coach the child to practice a set of activities until they're so automatic that he can fall back on these "self-regulatory habits" when he begins to feel disorganized and upset. Use role-playing and pretend-play. Children will find it easier to associate and choose appropriate behaviors if they practice first, as opposed to having to do it during stressful situations without practice. Practicing and teaching a repertoire of activities is helpful so that children don't get "stuck" when they feel poor regulation coming on. Providing charts with pictures and/or icons of activities may help children in distress build the bridge between their emotional state and the action that needs to be taken to mediate the emotional state, so they can return to feeling "in control" and balanced.

3. Children need immediate positive reinforcement when using self-regulation strategies. By choosing reinforcement that's meaningful to a specific child on his behavioral chart, behavioral shaping and reinforcement becomes more beneficial.

Emotional regulation strategies are embedded throughout the subsequent chapters. This is a basic area of difficulty that cuts across *all* SPD subtypes.

Self-Awareness Survey

The following survey contains a list of questions that can help provide more self-awareness in uncovering your own self-regulation mechanisms. The questions serve as a guide only.

1. What do you do to help keep yourself in a calm state? Write down three actions or efforts you use to maintain homeostasis (a balanced view) on a daily basis:

    A. _____

    _____

    B. _____

    _____

    C. _____

    _____

2. What types of sensory stimuli alter your feelings and emotional regulation? Are there things that make you feel better when you're upset or trigger a "down" feeling when you're doing fine?

    A. _____

    _____

    B _____

    _____

3. Do you have a repertoire (bag of tricks) that you are aware of that helps you feel balanced and in control (or at least somewhat better) when you're tired or when someone criticizes you?

    A. _____

    _____

    B. _____

    _____

4. Does it take you a long time to get back to a state of calm and feel that you're back in control when you get agitated? What helps you the most?

    A. _____

    _____

    B. _____

    _____

5.   Describe the strategies you use to return to homeostasis (a calm but alert state) if you are upset. Think about the following questions:

   A.   Are you the type of person who "talks" yourself through times of emotional difficulties?

   B.   Do you rely on "doing" and "being more physically involved" by using sensory input and motor output to bring yourself back to a balanced, calm state? Or, do you have other strategies that work to bring you back to a state of calm and balance?

   1. _____
   _____

   2. _____
   _____

6. Before you can deal with your own emotional regulation, you must identify the feelings that are associated with your dysregulated state. To do this, think about three times you felt that your emotions were not concordant with the situation at hand.

   1. _____
   _____

   2. _____
   _____

   3. _____
   _____

Now try to determine what triggered your response. Perhaps it was something that happened to you when you were a child, or perhaps it was something your parents would not have approved of but that you decided to do anyway. Perhaps it was just the stress of your everyday life.

_____
_____
_____
_____
_____

Activities to Regulate Your Emotional State

The following 10 exercises can help you and/or your child to regulate your emotional state. Try them and see which ones are the most calming and organizing for you.

1. Practice slow, deep breathing. Breathe in through your nose and out through gently pursed lips.

2. Wash your hands under cool water and continue with the slow breathing.

3. Massage the inside of your palms in a circular manner, making sure to include both palms.

4. Gently press the area above your top lip in a downward motion and hold until the count of 10.

5. Interlace your fingers and squeeze the palms of your hands together as tightly as you can, repeating five times until the count of six.

6. Begin massaging your ears, from the bottom of the ears toward the top. This is very calming to the nervous system, particularly when a slight amount of pressure is used.

7. Drink cold water through a straw with slow, small, repetitive sucks and swallows.

8. Stretch both hands and arms up as high as possible toward the sky, holding the stretch to the count of 10.

9. Apply essential body oils at the wrists, the back of the neck, and the temples. Try lavender, vanilla, and coconut, which are calming scents to most people. Olfactory (smell) sensations have a more direct route to the cortex of the brain and can sometimes induce a relaxed state quickly.

10. Find a corner of the room and gently wedge your back into the walls, as if you are being hugged. This also provides a quick, calming effect.

4

Sensory Modulation Disorder—Sensory Overresponsivity

Sensory modulation refers to the ability to adjust, regulate, limit, or enhance incoming sensory input. In a typically developing nervous system, the process of modulation occurs automatically, creating appropriate states of arousal required for attention, social relationships, memory, learning, and other key aspects of life.

Sensory modulation disorder is one of the three primary categories or patterns of SPD. Within sensory modulation disorder are subtypes that describe an atypical state of arousal and regulation, as well as unusual methods of processing sensory information. The first subtype is sensory overresponsivity, which is the focus of this chapter. Children with sensory overresponsivity may be too excited or overaroused to participate and engage in a productive manner. They are most often identified because they exhibit fight-or-flight responses to sensation. The second subtype, sensory underresponsivity, is the focus of the next chapter. In sensory underresponsivity, the child is too lethargic or unaware of internal and/or external sensory stimuli to engage and participate in a meaningful manner. The third subtype, sensory craving, which is discussed in chapter 6, refers to children who respond to sensory stimulation with behavior that is highly disorganized, with craving behaviors that appear to be geared toward trying to glean more and more sensation. Although the behaviors seen in the three subtypes differ dramatically, the three subtypes all have poor sensory modulation in common, which affects arousal regulation and behavioral responses to sensory input.

Many people liken sensory over- and underresponsivity to the gas tank of a car. This analogy is helpful to some people in understanding the difference between overresponsivity (children who respond too soon) and underresponsivity (children who respond only after excessive stimulation is provided).

The Fuel Tank Analogy

This analogy is sometimes cited to help people visualize what is occurring with the sensory overresponsive subtype and the sensory underresponsive subtype. As helpful as it can be in terms of a general association to what is happening in a child's brain, be aware that it is intended to be a simple explanation and not to have perfect neurological integrity. Most likely, the actual mechanisms of SPD will be quite complex, once they are known.

Like cars, nervous systems vary in size, the type of "fuel" needed, the quantity of "fuel" used for highest performance, and the amount of fuel needed to fill up the gas tank. Individuals' needs for sensory input can be compared to the varying needs of car engines. Think of the sensory input that our bodies need to function as if the sensory input were fuel for your car. The fuel (sensation) is sent to your brain through neural pathways, the way gasoline is pumped to your car's engine. Individuals need different amounts and types of "fuel" to function well **(Figure 4.1)**.

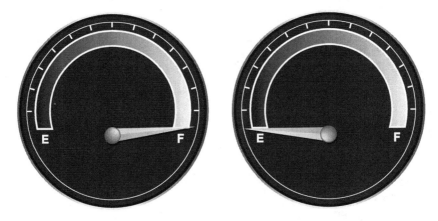

Figure 4.1. Modulation states for sensory overresponsivity (left) and sensory underresponsivity (right).

Some people have nervous systems that seem "more sensitive" and require less "fuel" to evoke an intense response. These individuals have "smaller gas tanks," so they "fill up" with only a little fuel. Often their tank fills so quickly and their capacity is so small that the "gas" overflows. This would be like a person who is sensory overresponsive, and the overflow might manifest as a temper tantrum or an aggressive or anxious event.

Individuals with small "gas tanks" become overloaded by sensation easily and often feel threatened, anxious, or worried. Children with sensory overre-sponsivity exhibit discomfort and/or fear from sensory stimulation that seems perfectly normal to typically developing children, such as a noisy cafeteria, a movie theater, or a sports arena.

In comparison, other people have nervous systems that seem "less sensi-tive" than others and require "more fuel" to function maximally or even to no-tice what is going on around them. The "gas tank" in individuals with sensory underresponsivity is deep and large and requires an enormous quantity of gas to reach a "full" state. When less than "full," an underresponsive child appears lethargic and/or unaware of his or her environment and the surrounding sen-sory messages.

So, the question is: How do we identify whether a child has a full or empty "gas tank," and what can we do to either "fill it" (if the child is underresponsive) or "empty it" so it doesn't overflow (if the child is overresponsive)?

This is the very question we hope to answer with this book. So let's roll our sleeves up—and jump right in.

What Is Sensory Modulation?

Our nervous system is built to automatically take in "just the right amount" of sensory information we need to survive and thrive in our environment. Built-in filters protect the brain from being bombarded by extraneous, irrelevant sensory input. The brain instantly alerts us if it senses danger that might affect our survival, such as a spider climbing up our arm, a snake in our path, or any other perceived danger. The filters in the brain regulate the amount and inten-sity of sensory information that the brain processes.

When we look at a tree, our brain puts millions of sensory stimuli to-gether (leaves, bark, branches, trunk) to be able to recognize the visual image of the tree. This recognition occurs without needing to look at specific, indi-vidual features of the tree. We discriminate only as much information as we need, and in most cases we don't need specific, detailed information about our surrounding environment. In the case of recognizing the tree, for example, the number of leaves on the tree is not relevant. Our brain automatically filters out the details to help us produce calm, ready-to-learn states, which occur during "optimal levels of arousal." We call these states *calm-alert states.*

In a crisis situation, however, it is normal for your arousal state to change, and you immediately become aware of more information in increasing detail. This huge increase in information can overload the brains of some children (and adults) because it requires extra energy and cognitive resources to deal with the new information. Your brain goes on high alert, as you have now detected the potential of danger. A part of your brain called the *sympathetic nervous system* puts you into this high-alert state as a protective mechanism, in case you have to respond quickly to avoid harm. Once the crisis is over, your *parasympathetic nervous system* helps you get back to a more calm and regulated state and regain your optimum state of arousal. We observe this process of stress and recovery numerous times a day in children who are developing typically. However, a child who takes in too much or too little sensory input or becomes disorganized with input is likely to have a sensory modulation disorder. Let's discuss the first kind—the child whose brain detects too much information.

What Is Sensory Overresponsivity?

There is a range of responses to sensation that is typically displayed within so-called *normally functioning* people in the general population. The variation in sensitivity to sensory stimuli includes differences in the amount, duration, or intensity of sensory stimuli that individuals can tolerate.

The level at which stimuli are detected is referred to as the *threshold* for noticing a particular sensation. We hypothesize that individuals with sensory overresponsivity have low thresholds and respond too quickly or too much to small amounts of stimulation. The result is problems in behavior, motor function, self-care, socialization, and other basic life roles and routines. This condition is sometimes referred to as *sensory defensiveness*. Individuals who have sensory overresponsivity are in a constant state of high alert, as if they're expecting danger or a disaster. Because they are on "high alert" (just in case they need to make a quick protective move), more information comes into their brain than is needed, which perpetuates a constant state of overload and anxiety. These sensory sensitivities often result in a desire to *fight, freeze,* or *flee* from the stimulation that is perceived as potentially dangerous.

Individuals with sensory overresponsivity are also hypothesized to have poor filtering of sensory signals and therefore have difficulty screening out extraneous stimulation from the environment. They may feel bombarded by sensory input, and their brains may perceive this sensory assault as potentially dangerous, even when it is not. Parents and teachers don't understand why they overreact to seemingly innocuous stimulation, but the behavioral outcomes are temper tantrums and meltdowns (often in public places) over seeming trifles.

Success in helping the child, teen, or adult with sensory overresponsivity depends on how well you understand what might be affecting him and causing his overreactive behavior, which is programmed deep in the nervous system as a protective device. Problem-solving to develop effective strategies for the child with sensory overresponsivity can be done by using A SECRET framework.

Symptoms and Behaviors in Sensory Overresponsivity

A child with sensory overresponsivity demonstrates behaviors related to anxiety, fear, mistrust, anger, withdrawal, and/or aggression. The child's world is aimed at self-protection, and he needs predictability and consistency to feel safe. Any change in routines, transitions between places, unusual settings, and people (especially strangers) can be enough to cause children with overresponsivity to freeze and shrink back, having frequent meltdowns and tantrums of long duration.

Sensitivities may exist in one, two, or all sensory domains. The most common symptoms are heightened tactile and auditory sensitivities, which often co-occur. Some children also have extreme sensitivity to moving their heads in space (movements that go in a direction against gravity, which are perceived by the vestibular system). In addition, a relatively small population of children also exhibits sensitivity to visual, olfactory (smell), and gustatory (taste) stimuli.

Notably, a child's behavior in school and at home may be different. This can be due to many differences, such as environmental differences or variations in how the children are treated in different settings. Sometimes we find that parents have learned to shield their overresponsive child from the daily travails that we all experience. But once the child reaches school age, he is no longer protected and is exposed to an array of sensory-enriched environments. This could trigger a fight-or-flight response and cause behaviors not seen at home. Children with auditory overresponsivity may "act out" and have meltdowns in music class, at a school assembly, or in any other loud environment, while children with tactile sensitivities may have difficulties engaging in art projects or standing in line with peers.

Let's go over some of the most common symptoms for children with sensory overresponsivity as it relates to each sensory domain.

Auditory domain.—A child with sensory overresponsivity may be extremely sensitive to sound and unable to tolerate high-frequency sound waves. When observed through a sensory lens, his previously random behaviors indicate that sound is uncomfortable and irritating to him. The symptoms of sensory overresponsivity in the auditory domain appear in **Table 4.1**.

Table 4.1. Symptoms of Sensory Overresponsivity in the Auditory Domain

Auditory Domain	Holds hands over ears to protect self from loud sounds
	Has difficulty completing work if background noise exists
	Is fearful of certain environmental sounds, such as a toilet flushing, dogs barking, vacuuming, using a hair dryer, and other infrequent but loud stimuli
	Fears movies or music concerts

Tactile domain.—In addition to protecting you from potential danger, the tactile sense provides information about the characteristics of objects. Children with sensory overresponsivity often miss out on obtaining precise and specific information about objects because they avoid touching things and can't tolerate being touched. Sometimes they appear cold, indifferent, and unaffectionate (for more information, see chapter 7 on sensory discrimination disorder). Children with sensory overresponsivity tend to respond best to sensory input that involves a heavy touch, as opposed to a light touch. They want to control the type and amount of sensory input they receive and are afraid of having touch imposed by an external source. Thus, they may shy away from being hugged but be able to actively hug another person if they initiate the contact.

Julie, a second-grader, comes to school every day wearing a loose dress with no underwear and no socks. Her teachers are concerned for her well-being and the social ramifications of Julie's refusal to wear anything other than a loose-fitting dress or floppy pants and an old, worn-out T-shirt, regardless of ambient temperature and seasons. She wears flip-flops and, upon entering the classroom, immediately throws her jacket (which she usually carries rather than wears) on the floor. She is anxious and irritable in class and can be extremely jumpy, as if she is in a constant state of alarm. Her behaviors resemble those of another girl in the class who experiences posttraumatic stress. The most common symptoms of sensory overresponsivity in the tactile domain are displayed in **Table 4.2**.

Table 4.2. Symptoms of Sensory Overresponsivity in the Tactile Domain

Tactile Domain	
	Is sensitive to certain fabrics (clothing, bedding)
	Complains about having hair brushed and cut, taking showers, and being gently kissed
	Avoids going barefoot, especially in grass or sand
	Becomes irritable with certain clothing textures, labels, and seams in socks and pants; avoids wearing new clothes
	Reacts negatively to textures on the hands, such as clay, finger paints, cookie crumbs, and dirt
	Prefers strong hugs; is very ticklish

Visual domain.—The visual system can forewarn and alert the nervous system to danger and unsafe situations, signaling the response to run, hide, hit, and fight. The motor responses the child makes depend on the stimulus and associations the child makes on the basis of past experience. In some children, mere exposure to fluorescent lights or bright sunshine is uncomfortable and can feel threatening. In sensory overresponsivity, responses to the intensity and duration of visual stimuli may be subtle, such as experiencing irritation when entering a room with fluorescent lights.

As Paul sits at his desk in class, he usually puts his head down, resting on his forearms. He blinks when he works on the computer and has difficulty making eye contact. He avoids being outside without wearing either a large cap or sunglasses. His behavior is so odd that other children have begun to notice it and make fun of him. The symptoms of visual overresponsivity are displayed in **Table 4.3**.

Table 4.3. Symptoms of Sensory Overresponsivity in the Visual Domain

Visual Domain	
	Prefers low light to bright light
	Squints or gets headaches
	Likes to wear hats or caps to protect his eyes from the sun
	Avoids or seems threatened by eye contact
	Is distracted or bothered by wall decorations or activity outside (as outside a window at school)

Taste/smell domain.—Children with sensory overresponsivity often have an array of food sensitivities, including overresponsivity to the texture, temperature, and/or smell of foods. This can make life difficult for both the family and the child at home, at school, and at friends' houses or when travelling. These children can become known as *picky eaters* who are difficult to satisfy. For some children, the picky eating can develop into problematic eating patterns and eventually lead to serious nutritional deficiencies.

Joy is a thin, frail third-grader who brings a bagged lunch to school every day. In her little Tupperware container is a small portion of plain pasta and butter sauce that she eats at room temperature. Her choices in food are limited, and she avoids texture, flavor, and temperature. She is one of the few children in class who doesn't like ice cream or burritos. Frequent symptoms of sensory overresponsivity in taste and/or smell are displayed in **Table 4.4.**

Table 4.4. Symptoms of Sensory Overresponsivity
in the Taste and Smell Domains

Taste and Smell Domain	Gags on textured food
	Avoids certain tastes/smells that are typically part of a child's diet
	Prefers extremes in temperature of foods—hot or cold
	Is overresponsive to odors in a restaurant or school cafeteria
	Does not like smells from objects that others around do not notice
	Refuses to go to the dentist, has poor dental hygiene, experiences discomfort when brushing teeth
	Is bothered by perfumed smells of lotion, soap, and shampoo

Vestibular domain.—Children with sensory overresponsivity in the movement domain can have several different types of sensitivity. The child with movement overresponsivity is terrified if her feet leave the stable ground, as when climbing a ladder or going down a slide. Another term you may hear for this type of problem is *gravitationally insecure.* These children avoid activities in which they have to jump, climb, or even perform simple motor skills, like turning a somersault. These fears lead to avoiding playgrounds, skating rinks, amusement parks, and any environment that has moving objects. These children may experience a terror of falling and getting hurt, even though any real safety risk is low. Another type of overresponsivity in the movement domain is the child who gets nauseated and somatically ill from movement. These children often get sick after an amusement park ride (it's normal for many adults to feel this way, but children usually do not).

Christian is crying and upset. His mom has signed him up for a gymnastics class, and the sight of the hanging ropes and parallel bars sends him into a meltdown. He spends the first few sessions sitting on the mat, avoiding any of the challenging activities that most children look forward to. When coaxed by his teacher to join the line, he waits with the other children but runs and hides behind his mother when it is his turn. The only activity he will try is getting into the pit full of foam pieces, where he would stay the whole time if allowed. Frequent symptoms of sensory overresponsivity in the vestibular domain are displayed in **Table 4.5**.

Table 4.5. Symptoms of Sensory Overresponsivity in the Movement (Vestibular) Domain

Movement (Vestibular) Domain	
	Becomes anxious or distressed when her feet leave the ground
	Avoids climbing or jumping
	Is fearful of going up and down stairs
	Avoids and dislikes elevators, escalators
	May avoid having her head tipped back when washing her hair
	Avoids playground equipment that requires movement, such as swings and slides
	May become anxious when moved by someone else, such as a teacher pushing her chair in toward her desk

Interoceptive domain.—This sense comprises receptors that sense the state of the internal organs. Interoception helps to regulate a child's body temperature and provides internal awareness of sensations from the heart, stomach, gastrointestinal tract, and respiratory and genitourinary systems and provides sensations such as pain, temperature, itch, hunger, and thirst.

Richard is a fourth-grader who has missed more school days than most of the other children in his grade. He has become increasingly more somatic throughout the years, complaining of headaches and stomachaches. He has problems regulating his body temperature and putting on and taking off his sweatshirt and alternates between sweating and being really cold. His toilet habits are a source of confusion to his teacher, as he spends more time in the bathroom than most of the other children. He visits the school nurse several times a week. Common symptoms of sensory overresponsivity in interoception are displayed in **Table 4.6.**

Table 4.6. Symptoms of Sensory Overresponsivity
in the Interoceptive Domain

Interoceptive Domain	Feels "stress" or worry inside her body as a body ache or pain
	Has frequent headaches, muscle aches, pains, and "owies"
	Ends up in the nurse's office at school often, with vague complaints of discomfort
	Is overly aware of sensations from the alimentary tract: nausea, severe hunger, fullness, and thirst

Principles of Intervention for Sensory Overresponsivity

Our approach is to teach parents the principles of treatment for sensory over-responsivity and to ask relevant questions, rather than prescribing *sensory diets* to remediate the disorder. Everyone is better off understanding the *purpose* of the intervention, so they can help problem-solve in situations that arise *in the moment*. The following five principles relate to the treatment of children who have sensory overresponsivity.

Principle 1: Normalize the child's arousal.

Children with sensory overresponsivity have nervous systems that are too quick to react or respond to various stimuli of low intensity. The key to intervention is using therapeutic activities to normalize the child's state of arousal. The child can be taught how to prevent himself from going into a state of over-arousal, in which he can't think or provide his own self-regulation strategies because his body is on "fight-or-flight" autopilot.

This occurs because some sensation has stimulated the sympathetic nervous system—a place in the brain called the *amygdala*—to respond. The amygdala forms and stores memories of negative emotional events. For example, if a child is repeatedly exposed to a sensory stimulus that he feels is aversive, *fear conditioning* will occur and be stored in the amygdala. At that point, negative associations with memories of that particular sensory stimulus are formed. These associations can cause future fear responses, even on just seeing the stimulus. The negative responses include fight (automatic aggressive response), freeze (immobility), and/or flight, with preparation of the body by increasing the heart rate and respiratory rate.

If a child has a tendency toward sensory overresponsivity, *slow-low* activities should help lower the child's arousal level. Providing ample time and opportunity for the child to become more trusting and tolerant of stimuli is also useful. Techniques such as massage, deep-touch stimulation, and vibration can help to achieve an optimal level of arousal. Once a child reaches a more "balanced" state, the more adverse sensory input will be better tolerated.

Principle 2: "Heavy work" helps to calm overarousal, especially when the child administers the sensation to him- or herself.

Children with sensory overresponsivity benefit from activities that require them to perform "heavy-work activities" to stimulate the proprioceptive system. Proprioceptive input is believed to provide calming and organizing stimuli to the nervous system when it is in an overaroused state, perhaps by overriding signals designed to warn the individual that danger is near. Proprioception derived from heavy work increases the sense of the position of body parts and perceiving when and where body parts are moving, which helps children to overcome sensitivity to movement in space.

"Heavy work" is a jargon term that refers to activities that provide deep pressure, vibration, and other kinds of deep proprioception to muscles and joints with slow but high-intensity input, such as that derived from carrying, lifting, pushing, pulling, and squeezing. Sweeping, mopping, shoveling, vacuuming, and gardening are great activities that incorporate heavy work. When heavy-work activities are provided within a natural, real context at home and/or school, the sensory input results in a meaningful and functional activity, enabling the child to organize the sensory input. Asking a child to use a small vacuum or broom after having a messy snack with friends or to sponge down a kitchen table after finger-painting helps the child organize sensations derived from meaningful heavy-work activities.

More examples of heavy-work activities are provided in the "Activities" section at the end of this chapter.

Principle 3: Predictability is king (or queen)!

Children with sensory overresponsivity don't like surprises. They need predictability to stay regulated and feel in control. Many parents and teachers have found that using visual schedules can assist greatly with predictability and, thus, with regulation. Some children even need miniature schedules to guide them through daily school and home routines. A mini-schedule breaks a difficult activity down into smaller steps—such as getting dressed in the morning, doing homework, accomplishing chores in the afternoon, and/or preparing for bedtime.

If the child with sensory overresponsivity is going to experience a transition and/or a change in schedule, providing warnings is critical. Preparation for transitions and changes in schedules can "make or break" a child in the moment of transition. "We'll be leaving in 10 minutes, honey," is the kind of preparatory remark that helps the child get ready for changes and transitions. "Let's count down together while we get everything we need to leave the house."

Principle 4: You must stay calm.

Inside your brain is a place called the amygdala, referred to in Principle 1. The amygdala (or amygdalae, the plural form of the word when discussing both sides of the brain) is a structure housed in the limbic lobe of the brain that controls emotion, rage, anger, and other intense emotional states **(Figure 4.2)**. Many people who have sensory modulation disorder have difficulty controlling and regulating emotions.

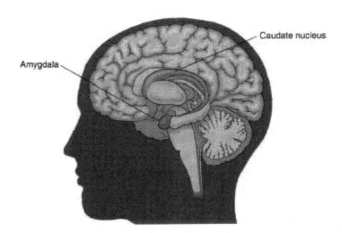

Figure 4.2. The location of the amygdala in the brain. Source: *scienceblogs.com*.

Never approach a child to talk to him about something he just did when you are functioning from *your* amygdala **(Figure 4.3)**. You will set yourself up for a power struggle if you go "amygdala to amygdala" with a child with modulation disorder, and in the end you will accomplish very little. Remember to choose the timing of your "battles" carefully with children who have sensory overresponsivity, and only discuss things when you are truly calm.

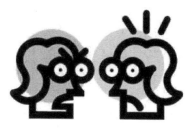

Figure 4.3. Don't go "amygdala to amygdala" with your child. It will get you nowhere.

> *Principle 5: Keep your child busy with predictable tasks when you are in public.*

When out in public, children's behaviors are often misunderstood by outsiders, who may be quick to judge your child (and you) and make negative, offensive, or unnecessary comments that can further offend both you and your child. Have games ready for your child to play so she is less focused on sensory experiences around her that may trigger a meltdown. You can play "I Spy" in line at the grocery store or sing "Bingo" in the car and even have your child unwrap several inexpensive "surprise" travel games during airplane rides. Refer to **Figure 4.4** for sample contents of sensory backpacks, which we offer to all parents at the STAR Center. This may get you started on the kinds of materials a child with sensory overresponsivity might benefit from having in his or her backpack. Changing things frequently in the backpack (but letting child know) is helpful for some children.

> *Principle 6: Avoid overstimulating sensory events at times, but slowly expose your child to normal sensations when possible.*

While sometimes necessary, avoidance of sensory stimulation in an effort to protect your child (if taken to the extreme) will ensure that your child will not grow to be comfortable in the real world. Noise-cancellation earphones are excellent when a child is trying to focus in the classroom. But if a child wears earphones all day long, he or she may never learn to adjust to background noise in the world without the earphones. Incremental exposure is better than complete avoidance of sensory stimulation. After all, our world is noisy. It has bright lights and lots of sharp edges. The goal is to teach our children to cope with sensations in a variety of environments that may not always be "comfortable" for them.

Josh's Story

Josh was a brilliant boy, who was 5 years old going on 35. He was referred to us because he couldn't get along with his classmates in school. He was the only child of a father who was a federal judge and a mother who was the CEO of a Fortune-500 company. He had many issues, but one was that whenever his kindergarten classroom got the least bit loud, he burst into tears and threw tantrums. After many weeks of treatment, his therapist finally had an opportunity to visit his home and school. The lightbulb went on!

His kindergarten was an open classroom. The children decided which station they wanted to work at and played there until a bell was rung, and they could either move or stay at that station. The kids were loud, and the teachers moved from station to station, encouraging cognitive and developmental growth.

The large, stately home where Josh lived couldn't have been more different. When we arrived, both his parents met us at the door. There was a two-story atrium in the entrance, and circular staircases wound up both sides of the large entryway. Josh was waiting at the top of the stairs. The house was completely quiet. "We like it quiet," his mom told us. "When we get home from a hectic day, our house is our haven. We can go to our studies and recover. Even Josh has his own quiet study where he can go to read his little books."

No wonder Josh was having trouble with his first experience at school! (He had been home with a nanny until then.) He was overresponsive to sensation to begin with, lacked auditory stimulation at home, and was overwhelmed by the "business" and noise of kindergarten. Among other things, we recommended that Josh begin to listen to music at home, starting at a very low volume and slowly increasing it over time.

Principle 7: Have sensory tools easily available, and teach your child to use them when you're not around.

An example of a useful tool is a *sensory backpack*, mentioned previously in Principle 5, which can be carried around whenever your child is not at home. We create a backpack for each sensory subtype that includes items to generate different types of sensory input. Children can self-regulate by taking along objects that are most beneficial for them. Examples of items to put in sensory backpacks for children with all three sensory modulation disorders are described in **Figure 4.4.**

Sensory Overresponsivity	Sensory Underresponsivity	Sensory Craving
Familiar items	Jangling, oddly shaped items	Heavy objects or items with moving parts that are interesting and goal related
Smooth items	Sticky and smellable items	Small hand weights, little gadgety games
Soft, squishy items	"Pokey" items	Drawing-type games to keep kids busy with Handheld computerized games

Figure 4.4. Sample Sensory Backpacks for Sensory Modulation Disorders

Use rewards to shape and reinforce self-regulation. Set up simple charts with appropriate rewards when children use their sensory backpacks independently for self-comfort. Meaningful rewards can be quite effective in changing behavior. We find that parents tend to use concrete objects for rewards, but remember that for many kids, the most valuable reward is time alone with a parent, doing something kid-oriented (such as going for ice cream with Mom or Dad on Saturday, with no siblings allowed).

Using A SECRET to Problem-Solve for Children with Sensory Overresponsivity

Remember our discussion of A SECRET in chapter 2? We used the letters of the acronym A SECRET as a cue to try to identify what might be done to help a child with a specific problem. Just as a reminder: *A* stands for *Attention; S* for *Sensation; E* for *Emotional regulation; C* for *Culture, Context,* or *Current Conditions; R* for *Relationship; E* for *Environment;* and *T* for *Task.* Let's use the example of going to the movies.

Jillian's Story

Eight-year-old Jillian has difficulty sitting and paying attention for any length of time. She is sensitive to a variety of sensations that she says make her feel like she wants to "run away and be alone." She typically doesn't have playdates, but today she has been invited to go to the movies with two other girls in her class. Her mother cringes, imagining how much of a struggle it might be for Jillian. Still, Jillian's mom is delighted that her daughter has been invited.

In Jillian's case, the challenge is staying "tuned in" and not "melting down" while going to the movies. Her short attention span could be a potential social impediment and could affect whether she gets invited to hang out with friends. Let's think about how we can use A SECRET to come up with strategies to engage Jillian's attention for the movie.

Problem-Solve Using T = Task

Cognitive behavioral strategies are great ways of reinforcing and shaping positive behavior. If Jillian's mother is worried that the movie date might be too big of a challenge, she could rent or download a movie of Jillian's choice and have a "practice session" at home first. She could also make a chart of small pieces of what the experience is likely to entail for Jillian, so that she can keep track of what she accomplishes and how many more pieces of the experience she has to go. For example, see **Table 4.7.**

Table 4.7. Sample Items for Jillian's Behavioral Chart

What to Expect	Yes	No
My friend's mom comes to pick me up and I go out and get in her car		
We get to the movie, get out of the car, and wait in line to buy our tickets		
We walk into the theater and either find seats first or buy popcorn and then find our seats		
We watch the short movies about what is coming		
I watch the show from 1 o'clock to 1:15		
I watch the show from 1:15 to 1:30		
(And so on until the end of the show at 2:15)		
(Then coming home is broken down into segments)		

On the day of the big event, Jillian's mother offers to take Jillian and her friends for ice cream afterward for a positive reward, if Jillian has a check mark in each "yes" box. (See **Table 4.8.**)

Now let's look at some other tasks that might affect attention for children with sensory overresponsivity. For homework completion or bedtime routines,

Table 4.8. Using Task to Increase Attention

Challenged Area	Elements from "A SECRET"						
	Attention	Sensation	Emotional Regulation	Culture/Context/ Current Conditions	Relationship	Environment	Task
Increased duration of attention at the movies							Mom treats Jillian and friends to ice cream after the movies

Table 4.9. Using Sensation to Increase Attention

Challenged Area	Elements from "A SECRET"						
	Attention	Sensation	Emotional Regulation	Culture/Context/ Current Conditions	Relationship	Environment	Task
Increased duration of attention at the movies		Use weight and pressure to calm Jillian during the movie					

"time timers" provide helpful visual cues regarding time. The timer pictured in **Figure 4.5** shows blocks of time against a colored background. As time passes, the "time timer" shows less and less red. When the red is gone, the time is up. This makes it easier for children to understand the passage of time. It can be used to organize how much time must be devoted to certain tasks at school or at home before the child gets a break and is also useful for myriad other purposes (see *timetimer.com*; available from *amazon.com* and many other Web locations). Another way to mark the passage of time and set time limits is to use a predetermined number of music tracks.

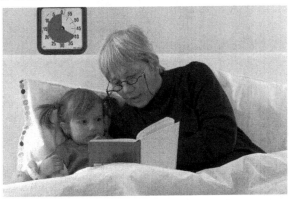

Figure 4.5. A time-timer can be used to regulate bedtime routines.

Problem-Solve Using S = Sensation: Weighted Items

Next, let's think about using sensation to help Jillian's ability to attend and increase the probability that she will be able to sit through the movie. Since Jillian has an overresponsive nervous system, sensation must be provided in a *low, slow* manner.

Weight and pressure can be used to calm children who respond to extremely low amounts of sensory stimuli. Overresponsive children become more balanced and less defensive when proprioceptive sensory experiences are used just before or during the event, such as right before Jillian goes to the movie. The use of various weighted items, like pressurized belts, socks, or vests (all of which may be found online—search the Web for "sensory therapy" and enter "heavy weight for treatment"), may be calming in a movie theater or classroom or at home **(Figure 4.6)**. It's best to use this sensory input before the stimulating event (in Jillian's case, before she goes to the movies), but some strategies can also be used nonobtrusively during the event, as well. (See **Table 4.9**.)

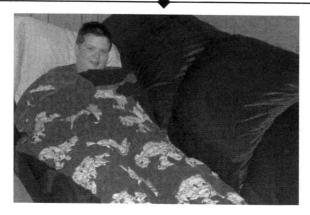

Figure 4.6. Use of a weighted blanket provides a calming effect.

Problem-Solve Using S = Sensation: A Sensory Backpack

Jillian can bring her sensory backpack with her in the car on the way to the movies. She can use any of the comforting sensory objects in her backpack to help reduce anxiety and/or any sensory discomfort. The ultimate goal is for Jillian to self-regulate, knowing what she needs to do when she's feeling overstimulated.

As we continue to think through Jillian's movie experience, we realize how much self-control she'll need to stay seated and not feel overwhelmed by her peers sitting close to her in the dark, with popcorn falling into her lap and other potentially aversive sensations that could lead to a "meltdown." Learning self-control is a crucial part of emotional regulation. (Just as a reminder, a child will be more comfortable doing a therapeutic activity that looks like something *anyone* would do.) The following compression-jacket activity provides proprioception in a covert manner.

Problem-Solve Using S = Sensation: A Compression Jacket

Jillian can use the compression-jacket trick at the movies. It is usually effective in providing calming input. The child in **Figure 4.7** has been taught to use the jacket to help keep himself in an emotionally regulated state. He places the jacket on the back of his chair, with his arms in the sleeves. The jacket is held firm by the back of the chair, providing him with a slight squeeze (proprioceptive input), which is organizing and calming. Hopefully, this type of input will help keep Jillian from feeling bombarded through touch receptors while sitting in close proximity to her friends in the theater.

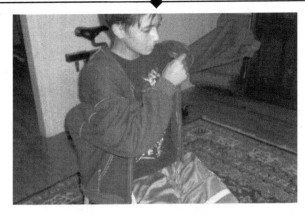

Figure 4.7. A weighted jacket placed on the chair provides pressure and muscle compression.

Jillian's mother can show her how to tie her sleeves around her shoulders and trunk, an exercise that also provides a hugging sensation loaded with proprioceptive sensory input. This strategy is helpful if the child needs to move around. In Jillian's case, this would be a useful method to use if she needs to leave her seat to use the bathroom or get a snack. The child in **Figure 4.8** has tied the sleeves of the jacket around his shoulders to provide calming proprioception. The tighter the sleeves can be tied, the better. This provides support for children like Jillian to be able to tolerate closer peer contact not only at the movies, but in many other situations where unanticipated touch and jostling occurs (such as while transitioning between classes in the hallways at school).

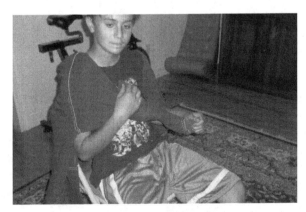

Figure 4.8. The sleeves of the weighted jacket can be tied around the shoulders to provide proprioception.

Table 4.10. Using Culture to Increase Attention

Challenged Area	Elements from "A SECRET"						
	Attention	Sensation	Emotional Regulation	Culture/Context/Current Conditions	Relationship	Environment	Task
Fear of not being regulated, alienating friends				Remind Jillian to do deep breathing exercises; chewing on popcorn may be helpful, as well as sending her with a keychain flashlight			

Table 4.11. Using Relationship to Affect Emotional Regulation

Challenged Area	Elements from "A SECRET"						
	Attention	Sensation	Emotional Regulation	Culture/Context/Current Conditions	Relationship	Environment	Task
Fear of becoming emotionally dysregulated during transition					Create a way for Jillian to contact you and go home if necessary; engage her in friendly conversation after the movie		

At age 8, Jillian desperately wants to have friends, but she's nervous about the upcoming movie date. She is worried that she won't be able to handle all the people, sounds, smells, and unexpected sensations that come up at the movies. Let's look at A SECRET and see if we can help Jillian work within the "culture" at the movie theater to make a modification that will help her maintain focus and not fall apart.

Problem-Solve Using C = Culture: Modify the Conditions

Theaters are dark and may be scary for a child with overresponsivity. Maybe you could give your child a small flashlight on a keychain that she can hold in her pocket for security. Practice deep-breathing exercises with her well in advance of the movie date. On the way to the theater, try more deep breathing to get her to relax. Let her know that she can use the breathing exercises anytime she feels worried or that she might lose control. Deep breathing is a way to self-regulate unnoticed in the theater and, hopefully, will also increase her focus on the movie. (See **Table 4.10.**)

Jillian may also want to buy some popcorn or candy to chew for oral-motor stimulation during the movie. We recommend getting to events like movies, birthday parties, and sports events early so your child doesn't have to deal with long lines. We also urge you to leave the venue after the exit rush.

Problem-Solve Using R = Relationship: Emotional Regulation

Let's review the elements of A SECRET that we could use to help Jillian. We've considered A, S, E, C, and T, so it's time to problem-solve by using the R (relationship) element to give us ideas. We know that children with sensory overresponsivity need predictability, because their world is often so disrupted and out of their control. Sensation can "hit them" anywhere at any time. Some places are more unpredictable than others. A child with over-responsivity needs warnings to prepare his or her nervous system. Perhaps you could loan Jillian your cell phone to call home if she feels like her senses are getting the best of her. The phone gives her the security of knowing that you can be there within 5 minutes to pick her up. (See **Table 4.11.**)

Problem-Solve Using E = Environment: "Time-in" Places

Children with sensory overresponsivity require what we like to call "time-in" (as opposed to time-out) places. "Time-in" refers to a place that a child can choose to go to self-regulate when she's feeling stressed or anticipating a sensory meltdown. Children feel safe and secure in small environments that are predictable and stay the same. In general, we recommend "time-in" places at home near the dinner table, in the family room, or wherever meltdowns are likely to occur. Small pup tents or large cardboard boxes make good "time-in" places.

Show Jillian how to make a small space by wedging herself into her seat sideways at the movies, with her jacket hood on. This small environment can provide some "time-in" for her if she begins to feel overwhelmed. (See **Table 4.12.**)

"Time-in" at home can occur in a crawl space under the stairs or in an unneeded closet. When a child is in her designated place, no one else is allowed to come in. She can stay as long as needed, uninterrupted and not bothered by family members or classmates. It is helpful if the space has some light weights to lift, a Theraband for stretching, fidget tools to fiddle with, and/or earphones to help quiet down the world. "Time-in" provides a time and place that's under the child's control to enable her to self-regulate whenever necessary. It's a place all her own, where her individual needs are honored. This is an environment for all children—not just those with sensory overresponsivity—to go whenever they feel overloaded or need a break **(Figure 4.9).**

Table 4.12. Environment Can Affect Emotional Regulation and Attention

Challenged Area	Elements from "A SECRET"					
	Attention	Sensation	Emotional Regulation	Culture/Context/ Current Conditions	Relationship	Environment	Task
Fear of not being regulated, alienating friends during the movie						Show Jillian how to make a little cave in case she needs some "alone time." She can turn sideways in her chair and put her jacket over her head.	

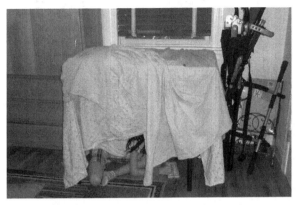

Figure 4.9. A "time-in" space can be created by placing a sheet over a table.

Problem-Solve Using E = Environment: "Push the Wall Down"

Another technique that involves use of the environment is teaching Jillian is to "push the wall down." Encourage her to find a corner of a spare room (maybe the ladies' room) and take a minute to push her back against two walls. This provides extra proprioception and increases her sense of safety and security, to help her feel safe and less overloaded. **Figure 4.10** shows a child using walls to provide herself with pressure when she needs it.

Methods like having "time-in" and pushing against walls in a corner cost nothing and are simple for children to understand. While cues may be needed,

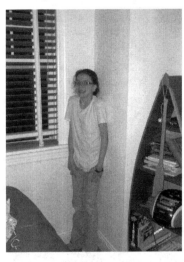

Figure 4.10. A child provides herself with pressure from two walls, which can be calming.

kids will take a big step toward self-regulation if they can seek out places of refuge rather than striking out, having a temper tantrum, or fleeing. Obviously, every child and every situation are different. There are a multitude of activities that you can use to soothe your child before or after she is feeling overaroused. Our goal is to show you how to use the problem-solving framework of A SE-CRET in a real-life situation. The strategies outlined here may have worked for Jillian, but they may not necessarily be useful for another child. *It's the thinking process that we're trying to convey here, not the specific activities!* You need to know how to think about and ask the right questions so you can figure out strategies that might be useful to your child at home or at school:

A = How can I use attention to help in this challenging situation?

S = How can I use sensation to help in this challenging situation?

E = How can I use emotional regulation to help in this challenging situation?

C = How can I use culture/context/current conditions to help in this challenging situation?

R = How can I use relationships to help in this challenging situation?

E = How can I use environment to help in this challenging situation?

T = How can I use task to help in this challenging situation?

When Problem-Solving Doesn't Work

Most likely, it will be difficult to do anything once your child reaches a full-blown temper tantrum or aggressive state. Of course, you need to keep your child and any other children present safe. If necessary, remove your child from the situation. Passively placing the child in a safe place where she can be left alone is often the best way to deal with full-scale emotional meltdowns. Try to be as unemotional as possible by saying, "I see you're having a hard time, Jillian. Let's put you in your special calm-down space [arranged ahead of time], and you can cry as long as you want to. I'll be right here to see you and play with you when you're ready to come out."

Table 4.13 offers some additional activity suggestions for children with sensory overresponsivity.

Table 4.13. Activity Suggestions for Sensory Overresponsivity

Sensory System with Overresponsivity	Activities
Auditory	Use a soft voice and short sentences, and DON'T TALK TOO MUCH!
	Listen to soft music with lower frequencies
	Use soft music, a white-noise machine, relaxing environmental sounds on CD with gentle ocean waves, etc
	Wear ear muffs, ear plugs
	Make noise-cancellation headphones or other headphones available, but do not force their use—it should be the child's choice
	Play "I Spy" while waiting in line
	Count down so the child knows when the next activity will begin, like going from the house to the car
Visual	Dim the lights
	Use natural light and avoid fluorescent lighting
	Leave the walls undecorated and use muted paint colors
	Wear a baseball cap with a big brim and/or sunglasses
	Use visual schedules to organize the child, especially when you know a difficult time is coming (if possible, insert your own photos into visual charts)
	Use a visual countdown cue, like a time-timer (see www.timetimer.com)

Gustatory (Taste)	Suck on fruit or ice pops
	Chew granola bars, fruit leather, or dried fruit
	Implement incremental exposure—at meal-time, start with an empty plate and add only one food to it at a time
Proprioceptive and Oral Proprioceptive	Use weighted objects, like weighted lap pillows, weighted blankets, and weighted stuffed animals
	Engage in isometric exercises, as in performing chair and wall push-ups
	Work out with weights
	Snack on chewy foods, chew gum, or blow whistles or bubbles
	Have your child help with a proprioceptive task when you are away from home, like pushing a shopping cart, loading cans of food into the cart, carrying the laundry, etc
	For deep pressure, wear pressure garments under the clothes, including Lycra and/or spandex garments; also, give firm hugs and massages
Olfactory (Smell)	Have the child select an aroma or fragrance to wear, like lavender, vanilla, or cinnamon
Tactile	Roll and/or wrap the child up in blankets and warm towels; for sleeping use cotton quilts and smooth sleeping bags; place pieces of soft fabric on pillowcases and use flannel sheets
	Take a warm bath
	Provide extra toweling-off after a bath
	Offer fidget toys, Koosh balls, silly putty, and bendable figures
Vestibular (Movement)	Have the child swing on a swing-set in a slow, linear motion
	Rock or glide in a chair with the child sitting in your lap

Interoceptive (Internal Sensations)	Use a hot water bottle for stomachaches
	Take a warm bath
	Eat soup and drink decaffeinated herbal teas, either hot or cold
	Apply ice to new bruises

Finally, here are some take-home points to remember with sensory over-responders:

- Remember that predictable activities and schedules are preferable.
- Try not to be in a hurry—take your time, and do what you need to do.
- Homework will go more smoothly if there are short, intense bursts of work, followed by a sensory activity; then, the child can do intense work again for a specific time period.
- Don't ask your child to "tell you about his day." If he can, he will.

Activities for Children with Sensory Overresponsivity

Activity 4A. Provide Comforting Sensory Input

In our opinion, no child should ever be forced to endure tactile stimulation that feels uncomfortable. In our view, "pushing the child through it" to make a neurological change related to tactile defensiveness isn't worth it. We do not want to add to the child's traumatic memories of touch. When a child becomes ready for various levels of tactile input, you'll be able to tell. We recommend that parents shop at inexpensive stores for paintbrushes, bath brushes, and other tactile materials that feel good to the child. A large fabric shop is a great place to find out what materials feel good. It is simple to let your child choose "special" material for a pillowcase, which can be made by sewing two simple seams in one piece of cloth (see **Figure 4.11**).

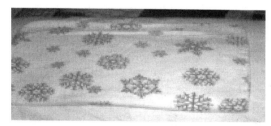

Figure 4.11. A completed pillowcase.

Purchase a piece of material that's about 4 inches longer than your child's pillow. Fold the rectangular piece approximately in half, with 4 to 6 inches leftover to tuck into the "pillowcase." Sew up the two sides. (Note: It's helpful to use washable material.)

The element of Sensation for the child with sensory overresponsivity can be addressed by allowing the child to keep a sport bottle with a straw on his or her desk **(Figure 4.12)**. This is one technique through which children can easily learn to be self-sufficient. Taking big swallows requires big breaths, which can be very satisfying and calming to children with overresponsivity.

Activity 4B. Heavy Work for the Mouth

Sucking is like a "heavy-work" activity for the mouth. Sometimes sucking thick foods like applesauce, yogurt, or pudding can be extremely calm-

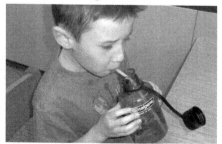

Figure 4.12. Drinking out of a sport bottle with a straw can be calming and satisfying for children with sensory overresponsivity.

ing for a child with sensory overresponsivity. Depending on temperature and consistency, the benefits can affect arousal and help provide calming and organized postural states for the child. Cold foods have more of an arousing affect then warmer ones.

Ice pops, hard candies, and gum—as well as other crunchy or chewy foods—provide a good way to affect arousal and can also be incorporated into self-regulation programs. Warm, sweet, and chewy foods generally have calming effects. Foods that provide more arousal include those that are crunchy, sour, salty, bitter, and cold.

Activity 4C. Incorporate Calming Stimulation into Daily Life Activities and Routines

Many calming games can be incorporated into bath time. For example, blowing bubbles is calming if children take a deep breath to blow. Warm water (as hot as tolerable) is also calming to most children. Some children find that certain olfactory stimuli (smells), such as lavender, have calming effects. Let the child choose an aroma that's pleasing.

Activity 4D. Heavy Work

The following list of activities can be used to enhance relationships between peers and families while helping a child benefit from the organized sensation of tactile input and proprioception. These activities can be done with the child to enhance the "readiness state" *(a)* prior to doing a task that may be difficult, *(b)* in between each individual step of a challenging task, or *(c)* following a difficult task. The activities described here use heavy work to provide a calming influence to a child who may be overresponsive to sensation.

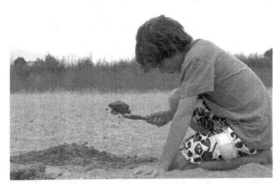

Sand

Note in **Figure 4.13** how playing in the sand causes a child to engage multiple muscles, especially if the sand is wet!

Figure 4.13. Shoveling and playing in the sand requires heavy work.

Gardening

Another excellent activity is gardening (see **Figure 4.14**). Digging, moving dirt, repotting soil, carrying gardening tools, and helping to transplant plants all make good use of muscles and joints and provide great proprioceptive input to calm children who tend to get overresponsive quickly. This would be a great activity for children to do before an overstimulating event, such as going to dinner with extended family.

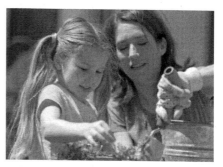

Figure 4.14. Planting and gardening can be a helpful proprioceptive activity.

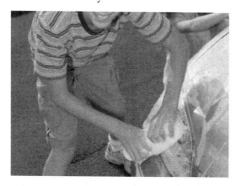

Figure 4.15. Washing a car with an industrial-sized sponge, soap, and water can be a good activity to do before a potentially overstimulating event.

Water Play

Most kids love to play in water, and water is actually quite heavy. The larger the sponge, the heavier it is. The bigger the bucket, the heavier it is. Using a little ingenuity, the parents of the boy in **Figure 4.15** have devised a "chore" that's both fun and therapeutic! This would be a wonderful activity to do right before an event that you know will be overstimulating, such as a birthday party.

Chores

Young children enjoy helping Mom and Dad around the house. Many chores require "heavy work," and the child will do them just to help you out. A girl carries laundry to her bedroom for heavy work in **Figure 4.16**.

Keeping in mind that your purpose is to calm down a child with sensory overresponsivity, what other household tasks might help your child lower his or her overall arousal level?

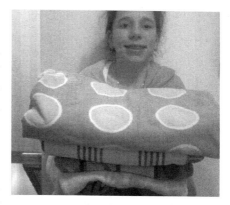

Figure 4.16. A girl carries laundry to her bedroom for heavy work.

Lap Pillows

Having children create their own weighted lap pillows is a helpful activity for kids with sensory overresponsivity. They can place the pillow on their shoulders, laps, stomachs, or feet to provide deep pressure (see **Figure 4.17**). Weighted lap pillows can be made out of a pillowcase stuffed with bags of beans, rice, and other grains (for children over 3 years of age). Another variation is to make sock snakes by putting beans, weights, or sand into a large sock that can be decorated with a face and worn over both shoulders.

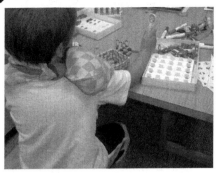

Figure 4.17. A homemade weighted lap pillow can be placed on a child's shoulders for calming input.

Activity 4E. Self-Directed Tactile Stimulation

Children with sensory overresponsivity do not want others to impose tactile input on them. They may, however, tolerate and even seek out tactile activities in which they are in control of the intensity and duration of the stimuli. Encourage touch input by offering a wide variety of possible tactile materials, such as brushes, vibrating toys, and the like. (See **Figure 4.18** for an example of what to keep in a tactile play box.)

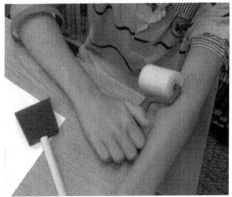

Figure 4.18. A sampling of items from a tactile play box.

5

Sensory Modulation Disorder— Sensory Underresponsivity

Sensory underresponsivity is the second type of sensory modulation disorder. The gas tank concept that was presented in chapter 4 can also be used when describing the modulation of an underresponsive child. In this case, imagine the tank is very large and needs premium fuel for an extra boost, an enormous amount of fuel, or frequent refueling to get the engine running.

As a general rule, children with sensory underresponsivity differ from typically developing children in that they require larger quantities of stimulation, a longer duration, and/or a greater intensity to be able to perceive sensory input. Intervention is designed to help arouse a child and make his perception of sensation occur more automatically and instantaneously. The goal is to have the child reach a "ready alert" state with an increased drive to play, explore, and engage with others. It is important to note that there is currently no physiologic research to confirm the supposition that these children have low arousal and perhaps high sensory thresholds. Although children with sensory underresponsivity exhibit behavior that is consistent with altered thresholds, no scientific research exists to date to confirm this hypothesis.

This chapter explores the issues that arise with underresponsive children and suggests ways to help increase their arousal level and "wake up" their senses.

Symptoms and Behaviors

Jennifer is an 11-year-old with sensory underresponsivity. As I watch her in a public middle-school classroom with 31 other students, I see that her eyes are open, and she appears awake. But when her teacher says, "Take out your history book and turn to page 52," Jennifer doesn't start to move until the buzz of children's voices and the overall state of the classroom environment become loud and stimulating. By then, everyone else is already on page 52, while Jennifer is glancing around at her classmates' desks to figure out which book to take out. By the time she finds the right book and the right page, she has missed about 10 minutes of what the teacher has said. If Jennifer remains in an underresponsive pattern with low arousal, she'll continue "tuning out" her environment and fall even further behind.

At her parent-teacher conference, Jennifer's teacher mentioned that Jennifer is inattentive and having a hard time keeping up with the class. In spite of Jennifer's very high intelligence level, the teacher suggested that she get outside help. Jennifer exhibits difficulties in the "big three S areas," including social participation, self-regulation, and self-esteem. Most of the other kids exclude her from their fast-paced games at recess, and she has been labeled as a "nerd." Without intensive redirecting, she seems lost and far away. Understandably, she gets frustrated and has frequent meltdowns and very low motivation, both academically and socially. Like so many underresponsive kids—particularly when they reach middle school and social interactions become the foundation of self-esteem—she feels unhappy and doomed.

Let's think about each of the eight sensory systems and ways to help Jennifer be more engaged and productive. The basic idea is quite simple. She needs stimulation, which we call the *fast-blast* type to differentiate it from the *low-slow* type that children with sensory overreponsivity need (see chapter 4), which means she needs intensive input in each sensory domain that is affected by sensory underresponsivity **(Figure 5.1)**.

SPD Subtype	Arousal Level	How Child Feels	Treatment
Sensory Overresponsive	Usually high	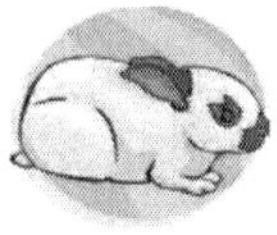	Use activities that are "Low/Slow"
Sensory Underresponsive	Usually low	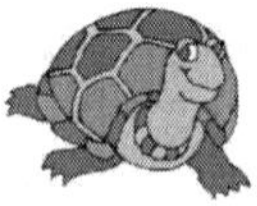	Use activities that are "Fast/Blast"

Figure 5.1. A depiction of arousal levels for sensory overresponsivity and underresponsivity.

No Longer A SECRET

Children with sensory underresponsivity seem to keep their thoughts and feelings "inside." They tend to get lost in a fantasy world that can seem almost like autism. (In fact, many of these children do come to us with a diagnosis of autism.) But if you can engage them, they come to life and exhibit intelligence and stability.

Ryan has sensory underresponsivity. His mother has to call his name five times before he stops focusing on his erector set and comes to the dinner table. "It's like he lives in a wetsuit, with all the accessories that go with it—the flippers, gloves, earplugs, goggles, and the neoprene skull cap!" she says. "By the time I finally get his attention, I'm exhausted!"

Ryan's mom is very perceptive. Children with sensory underresponsivity appear to exhibit a certain "numbness." Our goal in intervention is to increase Ryan's awareness of his environment by "poking holes" in his protective "skin" and waking up his senses.

Tables 5.1 through 5.7 suggest common symptoms that are observed in each sensory system if the child exhibits sensory underresponsivity in that system.

Table 5.1. Symptoms of Sensory Underresponsivity in the Auditory Domain

Auditory (Hearing)	Enjoys loud sounds and music in the background
	Has difficulty following directions, needs directions repeated
	May be nonresponsive when having his name called
	May produce his own sounds, hum, or talk to himself as he is completing tasks

Table 5.2. Symptoms of Sensory Underresponsivity in the Visual Domain

Visual	Has difficulty following a moving object, such as a ball, with his eyes
	May complain about having tired eyes
	Often loses his place while reading and copying information down (as off a blackboard)
	May write on a significant slant
	May seem oblivious to details of objects and the surrounding environment

Table 5.3. Symptoms of Sensory Underresponsivity
in the Taste and Smell Domains

Taste/Smell	May eat or drink something that is harmful without being aware of the smell and/or taste
	Usually does not notice odors and smells (which may also be a safety concern)
	Often doesn't notice or care whether food is spicy or bland

Table 5.4. Symptoms of Sensory Underresponsivity in the Movement/Vestibular Domain

Movement/ Vestibular	Does not experience pleasure or even a desire to explore his environment and move
	Displays a lack of participation in gym, sports, and playground activities
	Prefers sedentary activities, such as watching TV, using the computer, or sitting around
	Often has poor muscle tone and slow motor responses

Table 5.5. Symptoms of Sensory Underresponsivity in the Tactile Domain

Touch/ Tactile	Is not bothered by injuries, cuts, or bruises
	May not notice when he is bumped or pushed, unless the impact is severe or forceful
	Is indifferent to the feel of various fabrics in clothes (eg, cotton vs synthetic vs wool)

Table 5.6. Symptoms of Sensory Underresponsivity in the Interoceptive Domain

Interoception (Sensations in the Organs of the Body)	Has poor body awareness or body scheme
	Does not feel "stress" or worry inside his body, as in a body ache or pain
	Almost never has headaches or muscle aches and does not experience the pain of scrapes and bruises
	Is underaware of sensations from the alimentary tract: nausea, severe hunger, thirst, or overeating
	Is unaware of bowel movements and bladder sensations; often has "accidents"

Table 5.7. Symptoms of Sensory Underresponsivity
in the Proprioceptive Domain

Proprioception	Tends to slump or lean on walls, chairs, desks, and other furniture
	Uses too much or not enough force to meet everyday demands of activities
	Has difficulty keeping muscles working when maintaining a stable position
	Muscles are too weak to meet the demands of everyday tasks

Principles of Intervention for Sensory Underresponsivity

When working with children who have sensory underresponsivity, remember to incorporate the following principles into the treatment plans for those domains that are underresponsive.

Principle 1: Use alerting, fast, or intense sensory input to generate arousal.

Choose activities that are challenging, but make sure an adult is present to "scaffold" the performance of the child. "Scaffolding" means providing *just enough* support so that the child succeeds, but she still feels like she accomplished the task herself.

Listening to loud music with high frequencies is alerting. If you pair the music with movement, such as stomping the feet and marching in a big circle—which incorporate both the auditory and proprioceptive systems—you'll help enhance arousal in the nervous system and help the child make meaningful responses.

Principle 2: Use fast blasts of tactile, proprioceptive, and vestibular sensory input to alert whole-body responses.

Remember, "What you don't use, you lose." Children with sensory underresponsivity tend to sit around and not engage in motor activities (although they may play on computers for hours). The proverbial "couch potato" of yesteryear turned modern and became a "mouse potato," owing to the introduction of computer games.

Increase motor opportunities and demands as often as possible, while ensuring that the child succeeds. Replacing a chair with a stool, for example, requires children to recruit the use of the muscles in the back to keep themselves from falling over. Even more challenging is the use of a T-Stool, which balances on a thin piece of wood that is centered beneath the seat, as shown in **Figure 5.2**. This challenges a child's balance reactions and results in better posture.

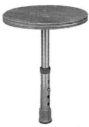

Figure 5.2. A type of T-stool.

At the park, increase sensory stimulation by jiggling the swing or challenging your child to bike up inclines. Ask him to wear a "heavy" backpack that has a water bottle, a snack, and a sweatshirt inside, and/or have him try jumping on a pogo stick.

 Principle 3: Use the stimulation of taste and smell to increase arousal.

Smell (olfactory input) quickly sends messages to the cortex (the center for higher-level brain functions) whenever a new stimulus is present. Scents such as menthol, eucalyptus, pine, and camphor can be powerful in increasing alertness. Have your child smell just a whiff on a Q-tip before he starts to do homework or have quiet-reading time. You may find a surprising increase in his ability to pay attention to the task at hand.

Certain foods can also be alerting, such as spicy chips, sour candy, gum, and bitter juice. If possible, work these items into your child's routine when he or she is most at risk of "tuning out," such as during quiet time at school **(Figure 5.3)**.

The sensations of smell and taste often combine while eating. Using a variety of smell sensations can arouse some children who aren't alert enough to eat and therefore demonstrate picky-eating tendencies. (See the Activities section at the end of this chapter for suggestions about making an "aroma bracelet," which will be available to the child all day whenever input is needed.)

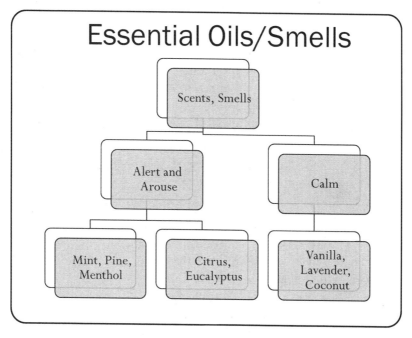

Figure 5.3. Using Scents and Smell to Elevate Arousal States

Principle 4: Use activities that are motivating.

A child with sensory underresponsivity is generally not interested in most activities that require effort and seems unmotivated to move around. Typically developing children, given an opportunity, tend to figure out some kind of movement-oriented game to play, like "tag." Thus, it is critical to get to know what the child *is* interested in and to design activities that take into account his or her personal interests. Whether it be Star Wars, Dora the Explorer, farm animals, the solar system, or whatever—you have to find out what your child's inner spark is.

Two activities that are motivating to most kids are popping bubble wrap and doing Focus Moves (from *S'cool Moves for Learning*, by Debra Wilson Heiberger).

Another technique that works for some children is inviting more active kids over for playdates. For children with sensory underresponsivity, being around more energetic children may naturally heighten their inner drive to play.

A SECRET for Sensory Underresponsivity

In chapter 4, we focused on using A SECRET framework to help a child with sensory overresponsivity sit through a movie with friends. In this chapter, we will take a more advanced approach to using A SECRET by choosing *strategies* to address the challenged state. This approach will give you a baseline methodology to think about. Because all children are different, the strategies must be tested with individual kids to find out if they are effective. Remember, the goal in this subtype is to help a child to *increase* arousal until a calm-alert state is reached. And the goal of A SECRET is to show you how to problem-solve to find solutions for your own child at home (as parents) or at school (as educators).

Judith's Challenges

When Judith was in first grade, her teacher labeled her as a "slow learner." Ironically, Judith completed some assignments at a level far above that of her classmates. The inconsistent quality of her schoolwork confused her teachers, parents, and therapists.

Now Judith is in second grade. Her teacher is aware that she has a tendency to "zone out" in class. In spite of her teacher's attempts to redirect her verbally, Judith has

Table 5.8. A SECRET Chart for Judith: Using Sensation to Increase Attention

Challenged Area	Elements from "A SECRET"						
	Attention	Sensation	Emotional Regulation	Culture/Context/ Current Conditions	Relationship	Environment	Task
Increase duration of attention in the classroom		Try following a Focus Moves chart by doing a series of sequential movements					

a hard time paying attention. We have chosen the element "S = Sensation" to create strategies to enhance Judith's attention level.

Activity 5A. Use Focus Moves to Enhance Attention

Ms Mooney, Judith's teacher, will use a series of sensorimotor activities called "Focus Moves" to help raise Judith's arousal level. This set of movement activities will be done right before Judith does her required reading. Focus Moves is a series of sequential motor movements, such as lifting up the hands, clapping, and jumping, that will increase not only Judith's arousal level, but also that of the other students in her class. Ms Mooney will try Focus Moves for 5 sequential days to determine if this is an effective strategy for Judith.

Figure 5.4 displays Judith's Focus Moves chart, with sequential icons for the intended movements.

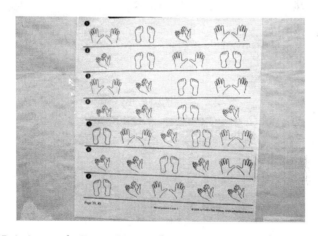

Figure 5.4. A sample Focus Moves chart: using sensorimotor activities to enhance attention.

In evaluating the effectiveness of this strategy, Ms Mooney told her occupational therapy consultant that the Focus Moves program worked partially, but Judith is still not able to maintain focus long enough to complete an entire reading or math lesson. Together, Ms Mooney and the occupational therapist choose to focus on "S = Sensation" again, but they decide to use a different strategy before starting with reading and math. All the children in class have been given small pieces of bubble wrap and will pop the bubbles to the beat of music. If Ms Mooney finds that Judith needs added arousal, she could ask the class to jump, balance, walk, run, and roll on bubble wrap—a sure way to "wake up" the nervous system! (See **Figure 5.5.**)

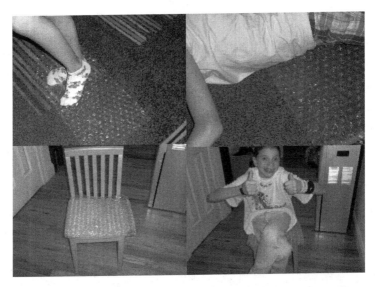

Figure 5.5. Sheets of bubble wrap can be used for jumping, rolling, and sitting on.

As Ms Mooney asks the students to take out their math books and turn to the chapter on subtraction, she overhears Judith mumbling, "I'm too dumb for this. I can't even find the stupid book. They should just put me back in first grade." Judith's self-esteem has been low since the beginning of the school year. Ms Mooney realizes that Judith's defeatism is going to keep her from learning any math today.

She thinks about A SECRET framework and decides to change the culture—or routine—of the class to try to help Judith feel like a "winner." Typically, the class copies problems out of the book and answers them on their own paper. But today, Ms Moody asks Judith to come to the blackboard to demonstrate how the problem should be set up on paper. Judith runs to the board, comes up with the right answer, and happily goes back to her seat to continue with the lesson. (To prevent Judith from possibly arriving at the wrong answer, her teacher could have given her the correct answer first and let her write it on the board for assistance.) Ms Mooney actually used two elements of A SECRET simultaneously in this strategy: She changed the classroom culture by using the blackboard instead of having Judith do the problem on paper, and she also enhanced Judith's emotional regulation by making her feel like a winner in front of the entire class.

Activity 5B. Use Smell to Enhance Emotional Regulation

An aroma bracelet can be worn by distracted, underresponsive children to help them focus on the task at hand. Making an "aroma bracelet" is a fun way to enhance children's attention and arousal states for learning in the classroom and/or home environment **(Figure 5.6)**. (See the Activities section at the end of the chapter for a complete description of the steps involved in making this bracelet.)

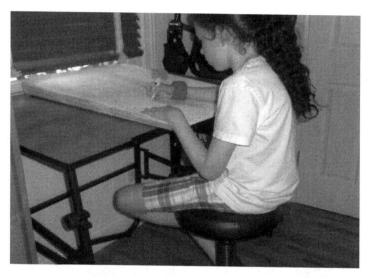

Figure 5.6. Wearing an "aroma bracelet" is a good way to increase arousal while doing schoolwork.

Activity 5C. Use Taste to Enhance Emotional Regulation and Social Participation

The gustatory sense can be used to affect emotional regulation (and social participation). Ms Mooney notices that Judith becomes lethargic and withdrawn as the day goes on. This pattern affects her relationships negatively. Judith usually feels left out, and her classmates feel like she ignores and snubs them. Ms Mooney uses the element of taste to try to build stronger relationships between Judith and her peers.

Ms Mooney calls Judith's mother and asks her to send a special snack for the class to share. Judith is allowed to go from desk to desk to serve the children the snack she brought in as reward for the entire class having focused on a particular lesson that day. The only condition, Ms Mooney says, is that all the children go to a new seat for snack time and talk to a classmate they don't know well. This seems to shake up the cliques a little bit, and she notices that Judith is chatting with kids with whom she usually doesn't interact.

Activity 5D. The Rolled-Jacket Strategy

During the unexpected snack time, Judith remembers to roll up her jacket and put it on the seat of her chair. (The rolled jacket [or sweater, sweatshirt, etc] on the chair in place of a cushion changes her postural state and ability to move, and the weight shift will help to enhance her arousal level.) Her occupational therapist has shown her how to rock back and forth on her jacket to keep up her arousal level up at school **(Figure 5.7)**. How great is that? Judith is self-regulating by changing her environment (the seat cushion) in the classroom. She feels much more responsive and happier in class. Everyone is thanking her! After all, she was the one who brought snacks for everyone to share.

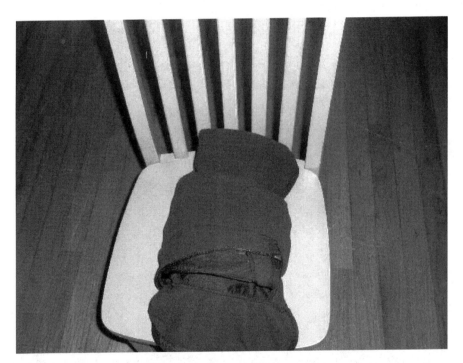

Figure 5.7. Placing a rolled jacket on the chair facilitates an increased arousal level, thereby allowing a child to focus more readily at school.

Activity 5E. Use Color to Enhance Attention

Children with sensory underresponsivity often have difficulty sustaining attention; when they are in underaroused states, they will sometimes perk up when they move to brightly lit environments. Just watch the faces and eyes of children when they walk past a tree covered in strings of colorful lights during the holiday season. They exude glee from the sensations that the visual system and the rest of the brain receive. Light affects our feelings of well-being, wonder, mood, comfort, and motivation.

Multiple articles extol the virtues of color, light, and dynamic motion on influencing attention and emotional states.[27-34] Look at our world of advertising and notice the color schemes that are used to portray messages to consumers. Something packaged in green symbolizes an organic, wholesome quality, and green is a noninvasive, calming color to the eye. Red is a color that instantly grabs our attention because it is one of the primary, intense colors that often increases our respiratory rate and blood pressure. In this way, color can be used as a visual cue for children to help with reading and attending. Some teachers tape colorful fabric streamers across the walls to keep children in the classroom alert. This may be too stimulating for children with visual overresponsivity, however, so it is important to maintain a balance between arousal and calmness. Some teachers arrange their room in segments, to be partly calming and partly arousing. Then they place the children who need calm or arousal in an appropriate part of the classroom.

To support Judith's attention level, let's modify her homework routine by placing red transparencies over her homework sheets. This may help Judith visually attend to the written details on her homework sheets. The color will enhance arousal, increase attention, and sustain focus, while providing added visual contrast to the words and numbers she needs to focus on to do her homework sheets.

Activity 5F. Use Alerting Sensory Input to Enhance Attention

Judith wears her aroma bracelet to help her sustain a more alert arousal state.

Remember that children with sensory underresponsivity benefit from sensory input that is fast and powerful. For the child with underresponsivity to be responsive and reactive, the sensations must be *alerting,* nonrhythmical, irregular, and unpredictable. All activities should be geared toward "waking up" the child's body and brain.

Exposing a child with sensory underresponsivity to full-body sensory activities that involve vestibular, tactile, and proprioceptive blasts (as a general rule) can be done prior to performing all tasks that call for sustained arousal and focus. Keep in mind that to create arousing vestibular input, the stimulation must vary. Simply spinning and spinning will not arouse a child. Shake it up! Proprioceptive stimulation is best if it is *phasic* (fast/short), so jumping on a pogo stick is better than climbing a long hill on a bike. Tactile input is more alerting if it involves light touch rather than deep pressure. By keeping all of these principles in mind, we can prevent a child with severe sensory underresponsivity from slipping down the slope into noninteraction and aloneness.

Table 5.9 provides some additional activity suggestions for children with sensory underresponsivity.

Table 5.9. Activity Suggestions for Sensory Underresponsivity

Sensory System with Underresponsivity	Activities
Auditory	Combine movement and music—fast and slow—in a rousing game of musical chairs Use a fast-paced metronome to play "Simon Says" Play "Simon," where you try to imitate patterns of sound sequences quickly
Visual	Brighten the lights if the room is dark Play "flashlight tag" (where you play "chase" with flashlight beams in a dark room) Find objects quickly in a darkened room with a flashlight Use fluorescent colors for clothes, toys, bedroom decor, etc Organize all kinds of timed tasks Use a "time-timer" for work completion
Gustatory (Taste)	Stimulate alertness with spicy, sweet, salty, or sour foods, including condiments
Proprioceptive	Apply deep pressure input that is quick (phasic) by using fast strokes Massage with a light touch and use alerting, smelly lotion Use bristly brushes and materials on the skin to provide a brushing type of stimulation in quick, light movements Play with vibrating toys Throw beanbags at targets; increase the challenge by varying the weight of the beanbags or tossing them at a moving target Hold the child's legs and have him perform a fast wheelbarrow movement, where he walks in a handstand position

Vestibular (Movement)	Swim and exercise in a pool by using fast movements
	Swim fast for short distances; try to get a personal best in a quicker time
	Swing in varying planes of movement (on the tummy, on the side, and upside-down) to provide different types of input; with the child's eyes closed, push him fast and then slow, having him guess if he's going slower or faster
	Introduce activities with unpredictable movements—run in a maze or pattern, skate fast, or ski in a fast or "tricky" way
	Use stools, crates, or other cost-effective objects to keep the child sitting in a more optimum state of arousal
	Jump on a trampoline while alternating positions (stand-sit-stand or stand-knees-stand)
	Sit and bounce on a therapy ball small enough so the child's feet touch the ground; use a "Hoppity-hop" ball and try to bounce it along a squiggly path!
	Transition between many positions (or different animal walks) while completing an obstacle course
Oral-Motor (Proprioceptive)	Provide crunchy snacks, pretzels, or vegetable sticks
	Offer hot, sour, sweet, and spicy gum
	Make hot or cold drinks and ice pops
	Suggest sucking on ice chips or crunching on a snow cone

Additional Activities for a Child with Sensory Underresponsivity

Smell (also known as olfactory input) sends a more direct message to the cortex (the center for higher-level brain functions) than other sensory stimuli. Many chemical stimulants can produce effects that are described as "hot, cold, or tingling." For example, sniffing menthol or eucalyptus can be helpful in arousing some children. Camphor can have a powerful effect, as it is even more aromatic.

For all of us, smell is what is called a "primal sense" because it's one of our oldest evolutionary senses. It permits simple organisms to mate, find food, and detect danger. Odor is one of the most important methods by which we communicate with our environment. It is useful to keep in mind that olfactory (smell) and gustatory (taste) sensations often combine during eating. Neurologic pathways for smell and taste connect with our emotional center and our long-term memories. Sometimes children who aren't aroused enough to eat well may be aided by the use of smell.

Smell sensations go directly to the olfactory cortex. Sometimes, intense feelings or memories can be evoked before a scent can even be identified. Smell affects a part of the brain called the *limbic system,* which is a primary center for emotions and memory. Sometimes olfactory input can be extremely effective with children who are sensory underresponsive. We adapt to smells relatively quickly (for example, if you smell perfume in a room, you can get used to it far more quickly than you could adapt to an annoying sound). This is called *olfactory fatigue,* and some scientists believe that inhibitory circuits in our brains may stop the olfactory signals from reaching our awareness.[35]

1. Make an "Aroma Bracelet" to Enhance Attention

Gather together some essential oils you think your child might like, and then ask the child to choose between two alerting fragrances. If the child likes a particular scent and seems alerted by it, use that scent to make an "aroma bracelet." Dab a piece of gauze with the preferred essential oil. Obtain a wide terrycloth sport band, and place the scented gauze on top of the center of the band. The gauze can be attached easily with a drop of glue or a double-sided piece of tape **(Figure 5.8.)**. Some children have skin allergies and can be allergic to having the oils on their skin, so always put the gauze on top of the band, away from the skin.

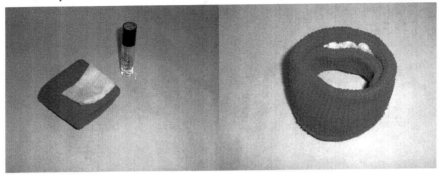

Figure 5.8. An "aroma bracelet" can be made out of a sport band, a length of gauze, and essential oil.

The beauty of the smell bracelet is that the essential oil stays localized to the gauze and doesn't disturb other people by permeating the room. By lifting the forearm up toward the nose throughout the day, the child can benefit from the arousing smell to keep him- or herself in a more alert, active state. Remember, every child is different, so take time to select a scent that he or she likes and finds alerting. The bracelets may also be effective while doing homework or tabletop activities to enhance attention levels.

2. Use Foods and Textures to Affect Attention/Arousal States

Using foods and textures can be an excellent, low-tech way to enhance arousal and alertness among children with sensory underresponsivity. Although many foods are chosen for their nutrients, some should be considered simply for their ability to help change arousal states. Crunchy foods, such as pretzels, chips, hard cookies, and vegetable sticks, are typically alerting and arousing. Chewy foods are thought to increase organization. For the child with sensory underresponsivity, food combinations that help alert and organize are usually the most beneficial.

3. Build Your Relationship with an Underresponsive Child

At home, eating with your child will strengthen your bond and relationship while bringing on changes in arousal. The family can sit together and eat crunchy foods, like toast, cereal without a lot of milk, and crispy fruits and vegetables. Crunchy foods are typically alerting and arousing. To aid in organization, try eating the cereal with cut fruit in it, like berries or dates. Granola can be crunchy if eaten alone or chewy after being soaked in milk. Since chewy foods are organizing, if an underresponsive child becomes too alert and seems disorganized, offering a chewy food might help.

4. Use Music to Enhance Attention

Incorporating lively music in the morning as part of an arousal technique can become part of a family's culture. As a parent, you might sing and dance to the beat of a favorite song as you awaken your child and start his or her day with a message to be alert and "ready to go" after a long night's sleep.

For underresponsive children who have many challenges with arousal states and difficulty getting themselves organized and together in the morning, try an alarm clock that plays CDs or an iPod to queue up favorite songs.

NOTES

6

Sensory Modulation Disorder—Sensory Craving

Sensory craving, the third subtype of sensory modulation disorder, differs from sensory overresponsiveness (chapter 4) and sensory underresponsiveness (chapter 5) in many ways. With overresponsiveness, evidence suggests that the functioning of the sympathetic nervous system differs significantly, with greater magnitude, more frequent responses, and less habituation to sensory input than is found in typically developing children.[36] It is logical to hypothesize that the opposite is true for underresponsiveness, but this has not been shown empirically in a large sample group.

Notably, the neurobiology that causes sensory craving has not yet been proposed. We believe that the three sensory modulation subtypes are based on different constructs. For each one, we think that behaviors can range from normal to significantly impaired, as shown in **Figure 6.1.**

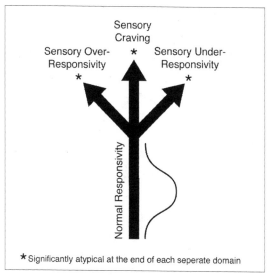

Figure 6.1. Sensory overresponsivity, sensory underresponsivity, and sensory craving are distinct entities.

What Is Sensory Craving?

As with sensory over- and underresponsivity, the fuel tank analogy is often used to describe sensory craving. Some have theorized that kids who crave (or seek) sensation have "fuel tanks" with perforations or leaks. This analogy stems from a seeming inability to become satiated, no matter how much sensory input is received. Typically, this behavior is observed in the domains of movement (vestibular system) and sensation in the muscles and joints (proprioceptive system), though it can be seen in other sensory domains, as well.

Following the gas tank theory, the sensory craver needs more and more "sensory fuel" to function, because no matter how much stimulation he or she gets, it's always "leaking out." Sensory cravers seem compelled to touch, smell, and lick and are oblivious to traditional boundaries and cultural mores (social manners and customs). They commonly flit from object to object or from task to task in wild, disorganized bursts of action.

Scottie is a 4-year-old who often seems out of control. His mother says he is "addicted" to sensory input. On the playground, he runs to the swing-set for vestibular stimulation but swings only a few seconds before he's off to see his friend on the monkey bars. He touches his friend's face and then darts over to the slide to smell the posts anchoring it to the ground. (He also smells other nonfood items, such as doorknobs.) In contrast to sensory over- and underresponsivity, the more stimulation Scottie gets, the more disorganized he becomes, and the more adamant he is about getting "more, more, more."

Even in this brief profile of a typical sensory craver, you can see how the "tank is not full" analogy falls short of the observed reality, because the more sensation Scottie receives, the stronger his drive becomes for even more stimulation—and *the less organized he becomes.*

Sensory cravers and sensory underresponders are often discussed as if they both have high sensory thresholds. Dr Winnie Dunn has developed a model that suggests that children who crave (or, to use her word, "seek") sensation need more opportunities to obtain sensory input.[37] Dunn further suggests that children who are sensory underresponsive benefit from greater intensity of sensory stimulation. We often see therapists in our mentoring program who interpret what Dunn has said to mean that both sensory underresponders and sensory cravers are not registering sensation and need more input.

We recently completed a study of 94 children at the Sensory Processing Disorder Foundation, in which we differentiated children with sensory craving from those with sensory underresponsivity by using a statistical technique called *cluster analysis.*[38] The purpose of cluster analysis is to determine if a distinct grouping occurs in sets of data. What we determined was that there were two *distinct* groups in the total sample of children with SPD—one group with sensory underresponsivity, and another, *completely nonoverlapping* group with sensory craving. Interestingly, both groups showed aspects of sensory overresponsivity, but the underresponsiveness and the sensory craving *did not overlap.* This empirical finding provides some support for questioning the theory proposed by Dr Dunn,[39] which suggests that both sensory cravers and sensory underresponders have high thresholds for detecting sensory stimuli (that is, they do not notice stimuli easily). Dunn's model postulates that the difference between sensory underresponsivity and sensory craving is that sensory cravers use an active strategy to self-regulate, while those with underresponsivity use a passive strategy.

In simpler terms, children with sensory craving display extreme overarousal with constant movement. They are in your face and in your space. Children with underresponsivity, on the other hand, are extremely underaroused, lethargic, and withdrawn. Given these enormous differences in behavior, it seems unlikely that the parts of the brain (mechanisms) involved with sensory underresponsiveness and sensory craving could be the same—or even similar.

These ideas have huge implications. The therapeutic recommendations for sensory craving are quite different than those for sensory underresponsiveness. Providing strong stimulation for a child with unresponsivity alerts him or her and is therefore desirable. Providing strong stimulation for a child with sensory craving is disorganizing and can be unwanted for both the child and others around him, as seen in Scottie's case.

In certain aspects, the behaviors of sensory cravers resemble those of children with attention-deficit/hyperactivity disorder (ADHD). In our research at the Sensory Processing Disorder Foundation, we are seeking psychophysiologic markers to distinguish children with ADHD from those with sensory craving. Our preliminary data suggest that many children with ADHD also have SPD.[40] In one study of more than 2,000 children who were selected to represent the U.S. population according to U.S. Census Bureau data (in terms of race, socioeconomic status, etc), we found that 40% of the sample had both ADHD and SPD symptoms, whereas about 30% had only ADHD symptoms, and about 30% had only SPD symptoms. Another study completed for a doctoral dissertation indicated that children with ADHD tend to have more impulsivity (called *response inhibition*) than their peers with SPD. On the other hand, children with sensory craving tend to have more difficulty adapting and adjusting to repeated sensory stimuli (called *sensory habituation*).[41] **Table 6.1** summarizes what was found in that preliminary study, in which children with SPD were compared with those with ADHD.

Table 6.1. Differences between Children with
ADHD and Those with SPD: Pilot Data

Parameter	Child with ADHD	Child with SPD
Inhibits responses (is not impulsive)	Demonstrates difficulty with inhibiting responses	Inhibits pretty well
Habituates to sensation	Habituates to sensation	Has difficulty habituating to sensation

Symptoms and Behaviors of Sensory Craving

Much like children with ADHD, sensory-craving kids demonstrate behaviors and drives that are often misunderstood by parents, teachers, and peers. They will touch, squeeze, chew, smell, bump into, and rub against all manner of animate and inanimate objects. Other overt, body-related behaviors may include excessive burping, flatulence, and noise-making with their mouths. (Just a side note: Many of these manifestations are related to ineffective interoception, or the sensations received from the child's internal organs.)

Behaviors like these aren't premeditated. They often seem unconscious for the child. Children with sensory craving can become aggressive and belligerent in their quest to obtain sensory input, often to the point that they're perceived as being "out of control." This quickly translates into a suggestion that the child is "bad." We see many sensory cravers who have been expelled from multiple preschools owing to combative, confrontational behavior. It's crucial, yet quite difficult, to help a child and his or her parents maintain high self-esteem when they hear over and over that he or she is a troublemaker.

Greg's Story

Greg craves sensation. He seems to get in trouble constantly at home and in school. He is driven to move his body and almost never makes it through his school day without getting at least one pink slip. He is bright, verbal, witty, and has a big heart—he's always the first to offer support to someone in need.

Greg's peers think he is "weird" and complain that he gets in their space. He seems to be unaware of boundaries, often reaching across his classmates' desks, bumping into them, and generally being "a pain."

His teacher, Miss Anderson, placed small pieces of tape on the sides of all the children's desks and told them not to cross the lines. When transitioning between classrooms, she asked each student to find one buddy and hold a small book between them to maintain personal boundaries. And, once in a while on the playground, she gives everyone a small hula-hoop, challenging her students not to impede on anyone else's space.

Miss Anderson's external cues are helpful for Greg. Over time, he begins to internalize appropriate boundaries, which in turn helps him begin to make and keep friends.

Children with sensory craving can be creative and innovative. Sometimes, when they are buddied up with other children who crave sensation, the collaboration can work perfectly because both children work at top speed and can get a large project done well. Children with sensory craving may also be paired with children who are sensory underresponsive, because the two subtypes tend to complement each other and balance each other out. Overresponsive kids may feel threatened and intruded upon by sensory cravers. Teachers need to be aware of sensory subtypes among students while making seating assignments in the classroom.

Children with sensory craving tend to be "thrill-seekers" who attempt all manner of dangerous activities as they strive to fill their needs for movement and proprioception and/or other sensations. Because their sensory craving may put them at risk, these kids require constant supervision. One of our moms described her son, at 3 years old, climbing up a tree so high that the fire department had to be called to help him down. Another mom tells the story of finding her 3-year-old on top of their new 7-foot jungle gym, yelling, "Look Mommy, I'm big!" This apparent compulsion toward recklessness only gets more dangerous as kids grow.

Alexander's Story

Alexander was precocious in achieving his motor milestones. He walked at 10 months, and by 12 months he began skating around the wood floors in his socks in his family's house. He intentionally crashed into walls, fell, got up, laughed, and crashed into another wall over and over again, stressing out his parents with his brutish horseplay.

Now, at age 8, Alexander enjoys the thrill of getting banged up on his junior-league hockey team. He has been to the emergency room five times in the past 6 months for open wounds, loose teeth, and miscellaneous injuries from being checked by other players. When asked if he gets hurt playing hockey, he replies, "No, never. I feel free, like I'm flying. I love it when one person falls, and we all fall on top of him. It's really crazy—it's awesome."

To live with a child with sensory craving can be quite chaotic and disruptive. Most parents, teachers, and siblings lose patience quickly, because sensory cravers are impulsive and don't seem to understand the consequences of their behavior, as illustrated by the following story about Sammy. In this story, you can see the good intentions of Connie, Sammy's mother, and her attempt to try to get her entire family involved in a project. Although Connie's efforts and attempts in organizing the family project were good, the outcome of the story shows how important follow-through and close supervision are for a child with sensory craving.

Sammy's Story

Connie is a single mother with four sons. Sammy, her youngest, exhibits sensory-craving behaviors. Connie struggles to manage Sammy and often keeps him physically close to her so that he doesn't get into trouble. One day in late fall, after Connie spent hours raking leaves for her sons to collect and bag, Sammy suddenly started jumping into her neat piles, undoing all of her hard work.

Connie and her other three sons were furious and frustrated by Sammy's behavior and seeming disregard for their efforts. Although Sammy apologized profusely, he seemed to not be able to stop himself from messing up more stuff in the yard. Less than a minute after saying he was sorry about the leaves, he headed toward a heap of branches that had been piled neatly by the garage. To the dismay of his mom and brothers, he undid an hour of their hard work.

Children with sensory craving often look for sensory opportunities in the proprioceptive, tactile, and vestibular domains (with the exception of children who have autism spectrum disorders who often seek olfactory, oral-motor, and visual input). Let's discuss behaviors and sensory symptoms for children with sensory craving, clustered by sensory domain.

Proprioceptive domain.—Children who crave proprioception enjoy activities that stretch and crunch their muscles through body position, weight bearing, and force. They are relentless in their search of constant input for the muscles and joints. Symptoms are described in **Table 6.2.**

Table 6.2. Symptoms of Proprioceptive Craving

Proprioceptive Craving	
	Is obsessed with excessive jumping, bumping, and crashing activities
	Loves to crack her knuckles, neck, and other joints
	Enjoys entering and crawling or squeezing through small places
	Is passionate about sleeping with multiple toys, stuffed animals, and blankets on the bed, leaving little room for her body
	Hugs, squeezes, and touches people and/or animals
	Habitually grinds her teeth
	Likes tight-fitting clothes
	Is unruly, as she craves and gets input no matter where she is
	Loves hanging from bars on the playground or doing other climbing and stretching activities

Vestibular domain.—Children who crave vestibular stimulation love movement in all directions and angles. They jump, climb, skip, roll, and do whatever they can to move in all planes of space. When they are moving, their moods are often cheerful and their actions vigorous. Symptoms are described in **Table 6.3.**

Table 6.3. Symptoms of Vestibular Craving

Vestibular Craving	Frequently falls on the floor and rolls around intentionally
	Insists on intense movement input, such as flipping, turning, rotating, and being inverted; can spin for a long time without getting dizzy
	Is adamant about roughhousing, play fighting, and being tossed in the air
	Jumps on beds and couches aggressively
	Loves extreme fast-moving input, such as ice-skating, skiing, sledding, bike-riding, rollerblading, skateboarding, motorcycling, speedboating, racing cars, hitting road bumps, and riding roller coasters and other amusement park rides; may grow up to be an "extreme" athlete, if coordinated enough
	Is not calmed down by additional movement input; tends to get more aroused and disorganized as movement increases

Tactile domain.—Children who crave tactile sensation can seem intrusive in the way they touch people and objects. Textures and surfaces are explored repeatedly though touching, squeezing, licking, and other forms of tactile-craving behaviors. Tactile-craving behaviors are listed in **Table 6.4**.

Table 6.4. Symptoms of Tactile Craving

Tactile Craving	Needs to constantly touch surfaces and textures, particularly soft and cuddly objects
	May cause others discomfort and a sense of violation of personal space with the need to touch
	Frequently bumps into objects and people
	Wants to play with messy stimuli for long periods of time
	May mouth or bite objects beyond the appropriate developmental stages
	May rub or bite the skin

No Longer A SECRET

Oral-motor, olfactory, and gustatory domains.—Oral sensation (which is often proprioceptive) may provide intense stimulation when the mouth muscles and joints are involved. Some children who need oral-motor stimulation can be uncontrollable and challenging until they get their oral-motor "fix." Often they provide their own input by chewing on their shirt sleeves, hair, or pencils.

Typically (but not always), children with sensory craving and developmental delays use smell as a way to learn about objects and people. Exploring the qualities of inanimate objects by licking them may be noted in a child who tastes walls, books, teachers, peers, and pets. The symptoms of oral-motor, olfactory, and gustatory craving are described in **Table 6.5**.

Table 6.5. Symptoms of Oral-Motor, Olfactory, and Gustatory Craving

Oral–Motor, Olfactory, and Gustatory Craving	
	Licks or chews strands of hair
	Smells people, animals, and objects
	Licks objects, people, and foods (prior to tasting)
	Bites rather than sucks candies, unless cued
	Has a constant desire for chewing gum, if allowed
	Desires crunchy foods like chips, pretzels, and cookies
	Often particularly likes one type of food: sweet, sour, and/or salty
	Bites on sleeves, pencil erasers, paper clips; always has something in his or her mouth

Visual domain.—Children with visual craving love and seek out visual stimulation to an excessive degree. In today's digital age, these kids have many opportunities to glean this input through television, videos, computers, and other forms of two-dimensional (often stationary) input. Children with sensory craving may overindulge in this type of input, become overfocused on the visual stimulation, and seem unable to attend to other important sensory information around them. Sitting in front of a television watching bright lights, fluorescent colors, or static waves may be more engaging than listening to their parents. Picking up small particles on the classroom carpet may be more fascinating than attending to the book being read by the teacher. The child with visual craving may become lost in visual details and miss the "whole" picture. See **Table 6.6** for symptoms of visual craving.

Table 6.6. Symptoms of Visual Craving

Visual Craving	Is attracted to watching flickering lights or nonmeaningful visual stimuli
	Tends to choose objects that are brightly colored
	Is captivated by and can spend hours in front of a television, computer, or video game
	Gazes at spinning objects for long periods of time
	Attends to one visual detail for a long time, such as a single page of a book, the tire of a car, or a blackboard

Auditory domain.—Children who crave input in the auditory domain seek unreasonably loud auditory stimuli, can't control their voices or noise-making, and are often the loudest kids in the classroom. Symptoms related to auditory craving are displayed in **Table 6.7.**

Table 6.7. Symptoms of Auditory Craving

Auditory Craving	Prefers the volume on televisions and music at a level that is uncomfortably loud for others
	Uses a loud voice—possibly almost a shouting level—when speaking
	Tends to make noises in the background while doing other tasks
	Enjoys noisy environments, such as sports arenas and malls

Principles of Intervention for Sensory Craving

The use of appropriate principles of intervention is critical in supporting sensory-craving kids. The following eight principles serve as guidelines for teachers, parents, and therapists. The guidelines help sensory cravers to organize sensation, direct their actions, and stop annoying the people around them. Many of these strategies are also useful for children with ADHD.

> ### Principle 1: Create organized movement experiences that are goal-directed and purposeful.

Whenever possible, connect movement such as running, jumping, and hopping to a specific goal. Remember how disorganized Scottie became after running, "just to run"? Creating a relay-race activity on the soccer field is a beneficial activity, as long as it is set up in a sequential, purposeful manner that helps the child to organize the sensation of running. Pair gross-motor activities with goals. Rolling or hopping activities can be set up so that children pick up puzzle pieces in the direction in which they roll. Have the children pick up the pieces one at a time, until all the pieces are collected and the puzzle is complete. With activities that are structured, planned, and purposeful, children with sensory craving experience a higher degree of sensory organization.

Anthony and Amy

Miss Grace is a new kindergarten teacher, with a background in special education. One of her students, Anthony, has many sensory-craving symptoms.

Anthony is a bundle of energy, is always in motion, and is unable to sit and attend properly in class. To calm him down, Miss Grace pairs vestibular or proprioceptive sensation with sequential movements that have a purpose. For example, she created a maze that starts with the spinning chair at her desk. Each child gets one spin in each direction (to increase arousal) and then has to search for puzzle pieces that match his or her assigned topic (each pair of kids has been asked to find puzzle pieces for one of the United States). The puzzle pieces are located at every main intersection of the maze. The children have to move over, under, and around chairs to get through the maze to find their puzzle pieces.

Anthony was buddied with Amy, a quiet but determined little girl who helped him stay focused. Anthony brought speed and energy to this goal-oriented activity, and starting the task with a small but organized amount of vestibular stimulation helped Anthony stay on task and follow directions. He showed more focus and self-direction and better self-regulation than usual. This kind of structured task also helped him to stay within the framework of "good" behavior. Together, Anthony and Amy completed the maze and found all the puzzle pieces first! Buddying the "right" pairs took Miss Grace some time to work out for the whole class, but it was definitely worth it. Everyone now had his or her "project buddy" for the month.

Principle 2: Use intermittent, varying, or interrupted vestibular input.

Children with sensory craving will organize sensation better when activities provide movement that stops and starts unexpectedly. It's also helpful to make sure that the child's head isn't upright. For example, set up activities in which he spins for 5 seconds, then spins the other way for 5 seconds, then switches to jumping and swinging, each for 5-second intervals so that his head leans in varying directions. This channels the overwhelming drive to keep moving so he can "stay with" an organized activity.

Sensory seekers often habituate to constant movement. For example, an ice-skater doing rapid spins does not feel the turns like you or I would. Her brain has learned to suppress the sensation of spinning. Unless you can "change it up" by doing an activity that stops and starts—or one in which the child's head is not in an upright position—he or she hardly registers the movement. Moving in ways that tilt the head in different directions provides strong input to the vestibular system. Instead of not feeling the movement, the child may feel it much more intensely (possibly so much that he or she can only stay in that position for a short period of time).

When working with a child who craves constant movement, DO NOT spin them, swing them wildly, or have them jump or bounce for long periods of time. Involve them in games like "Duck-Duck-Goose," "Musical Chairs," and "Red Light/Green Light," or other activities that provide only intermittent movement stimulation. Continuous activity, especially movement, is part of the sensory-craving child's daily repertoire. Use cognitive behavioral approaches to teach the child "STOP," so he or she can voluntarily "turn off" and stop after being in motion. Play stop-and-go games with stop signs, stoplights, and flash cards. All children can use a boost of "stop" skills; honing those skills in a game is much more fun than reminding children to hold still over and over again. This is a skill that takes practice for children with sensory craving, and when they begin to control their own behavior, they can stop bouncing off the walls and focus on their true gifts.

Principle 3: Use programs that incorporate "heavy work"—purposeful tasks with proprioceptive components.

The "best" proprioceptive input is based on natural "heavy work" activities at home and at school. Assigned, goal-directed heavy work in a classroom (such as washing and wiping down tables after painting, sweeping after art or snack time, or placing all the chairs onto the desks at the end of the day) provides structure while incorporating proprioception. Additional examples of heavy work are provided at the end of chapter 4, our chapter on sensory overresponsiveness, because sensory overresponsive children also benefit from heavy-work activities (though for a different reason). With sensory overresponsivity, heavy work is calming to a nervous system that is ready to go into fight-or-flight mode. With sensory craving, heavy work provides an alternative to constant motion, and the proprioception is organizing or regulating to the sensory-driven child. Isometric exercises and weight-lifting with 1- to 5-pound weights are examples of goal-directed heavy work that is fun for older kids and can be done with a parent before school to start the day in a more regulated manner.

This type of sensory input is also beneficial after a long day at school, before doing homework, and on the weekends when there is less structure and organization. Jobs and chores assigned by parents or teachers should be short and fun, so a child can be successful. Children with sensory craving can even select or create their own heavy-work tasks that they find interesting. Socks filled with sand and beans and small hand weights can be placed inside a sensory backpack and used independently as part of a self-regulation program to help organize children who crave sensation.

Principle 4: Use environmental modifications when socializing with peers.

Simple modifications (such as placing tape on either side of a child's desk that no one else is allowed to cross over or using stickers to differentiate spatial boundaries and personal space) can make an enormous difference in the way children with sensory craving perceive their own and others' personal space. Not getting into other peoples' faces and spaces can make a huge difference in being accepted by peers.

Principle 5: Use enclosed or small spaces to control activity.

Open, large spaces invite trouble and mischief for children with sensory craving. Taking a child to a busy mall, an airport, or a grocery store is a sure way of creating sensory disorganization, especially if running and aimless behavior are part of the event. Bring along a sensory backpack so the child has tools he or she has selected and practiced to enhance self-regulation.

A SECRET for Sensory Craving

A SECRET framework for the sensory-craving child can help the teacher, parent, or therapist create effective "on the spot" plans that address the child's challenges. These challenges can be seen during a required task or in a particular environment. If you *consider all elements* and choose the one or two you think will work best from A SECRET—attention, sensation, emotional regulation, culture and current conditions, relationships, environment, and task—success will be maximized.

Tommy's Story

Seven-year-old Tommy has sensory craving. He is in first grade and receives occupational therapy twice a week with in-classroom services. One of the objectives for Tommy includes helping him work independently and complete fine-motor tasks in class.

Today, the students are working independently to complete a project that includes coloring and cutting out pictures of favorite animals. The children are also required to write a few short sentences about ways that they are like the animal they have chosen. Although Tommy is capable of completing this task, he is already distracted by what Audrey, the child sitting next to him, is doing and needs a lot of redirecting and refocusing. Louise, Tommy's occupational therapist, is trying to help Tommy with the goal of increasing focus and concentration and will use A SECRET framework within the classroom to help Tommy stay focused without being impulsive and getting into trouble.

Attention is the challenged area about which Louise has been asked to consult.

Problem-Solve Using S = Sensation to Affect Attention

This is the first strategy Louise decides to consider. Louise has chosen to use the element of sensation to address Tommy's distraction. Her plan is to bring a variety of functional fidget tools to offer Tommy (see the end of the chapter for a complete description of functional fidget tools and guidelines for choosing them). These are small, nondistracting items that help him attend and focus on his own work, as opposed to being distracted by the peers around him **(Figure 6.2)**. She tries common, little "everyday" items like pen tops, paper clips, erasers, and pencil grips. She finds that, for some reason, a pen top works especially well for Tommy, who fidgets with it while listening to his teacher's directions. We find that the best functional fidget tools are common items with limited sensory properties, so that the child can attend without becoming distracted.

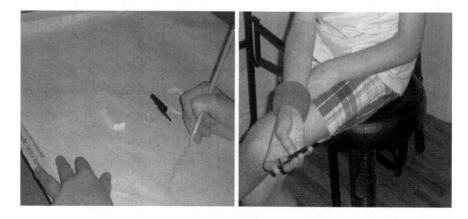

Figure 6.2. Functional fidget tools.

Louise notes that Tommy picks up the fidget tool, puts it in his hand, and starts to flip through a magazine with his other hand. He is looking for pictures of animals for his project. She sees him wiggling around in his seat, obviously wanting to move. She knows that sitting in one place is hard for him and that momentarily, he will be getting up to dart around the room. To avoid this, Louise needs to introduce a different kind of sensation so that Tommy's craving to move will be supplanted by something stronger.

Is there another way that sensation can be used to increase attention? Louise decides to try the "rolled jacket" activity.

Organized opportunities for almost any sensory experience are usually helpful for a child with sensory-craving behaviors. Small movements can be particularly helpful. The rolled-jacket activity provides movement and weight-shifting for Tommy in the classroom, while allowing him to attend and remain focused on his project. Louise shows Tommy how to roll up his sweatshirt and sit on it **(Figure 6.3)**. She has made a functional "sit-disk" facsimile. Tommy is thrilled about being given the opportunity to move in his seat. He is especially happy that he doesn't have to use some conspicuous piece of therapeutic equipment that sets him apart from other kids. Some of the other kids have even incorporated the same self-regulation strategy when they need movement.

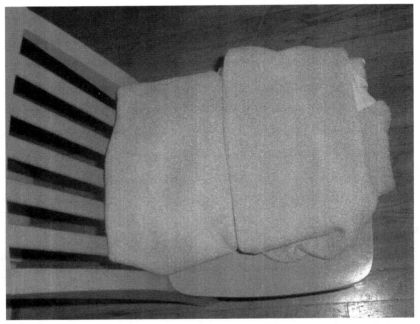

Figure 6.3. Using a rolled jacket on a chair helps a child be able to move in his seat without having to buy an inflatable disk.

Tommy is now doing better, slowly shifting his weight back and forth in his seat while choosing pictures of puppies and birds in his magazine. Louise is thrilled and wants to reinforce Tommy's great focus to his task. She chooses to use the element of emotional regulation to keep him on track. She thinks about what she knows about Tommy and what he might feel is really a positive reward.

Emotional regulation is now the area that Louise wants to focus on.

Problem-Solve Using T = Task to Affect Emotional Regulation

Louise quickly draws a little chart with boxes that constitute the steps of the animal project assigned by his teacher. She has already placed two stickers on the chart, so Tommy is partway there without trying! He is getting ready to cut out the puppy and bird he has chosen for his project. He knows that once he gets 10 stickers, he may choose a little toy from the treasure box in Louise's therapy room.

A SECRET has many dimensions. It's designed so that if your first strategy doesn't work or if you need to continue to support the child during the task, you can scan (or think) horizontally across the concepts that make up the acronym "A SECRET" and pick another element to try. So, if the sticker strategy didn't help Tommy stay focused and on task, Louise or Tommy's teacher or parent would choose another element to help with his challenged area. For example, Louise could have used scented stickers in flavors that Tommy likes the most (such as vanilla, bubble gum, chocolate chip cookies, or cinnamon). The calming smells on the stickers could aid in Tommy's emotional regulation and encourage him to focus on the task at hand.

Louise and Ms Zinn, Tommy's teacher, are proud of his progress in following the directions of the task he is working on. Unfortunately, many of the students are taking a long time to finish up. Now, nearly 20 minutes into the activity, Tommy is getting fidgety and antsy again. Ms Zinn is an open-minded teacher and has decided to change the culture in her classroom to help Tommy finish his activity. Instead of sitting straightforward in their seats, she suggests that the students use Chair Moves, a program of five chair positions that provides changing sensations while staying in one's seat.

Task is now the challenged area in which Ms Zinn wants to support Tommy.

Problem-Solve Using C = Culture to Affect Task Completion

Ms Zinn has posted pictures of the five Chair Moves positions on the wall for the children to see. Of the five positions, Tommy chooses position 1 in the Chair Moves sequence and places his chair so that the back of it faces his desk while he straddles the chair **(Figure 6.4)**. Tommy sits without back support and uses his core strength to sit upright. Movement and proprioception are inherent to this position and help change his arousal state.

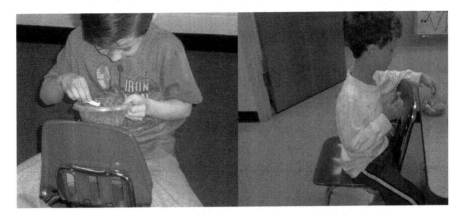

Figure 6.4. Chair Moves position 1 involves straddling the chair backward, using the core strength to sit up without having back support.

This position works for Tommy for a few minutes. But Louise sees that Tommy is starting to talk to his neighbors and look over the shoulder of Audrey, who is sitting next to him. She asks if Tommy can think of another thing he can do to stay focused on the task. Louise is trying to increase his independence level and awareness of when he needs to switch to a new strategy. Tommy decides to try position 2 of Chair Moves. Since Louise can see that Tommy is well on his way to interrupting Audrey, she begins to consider the element of *relationship* in A SECRET. As Tommy turns his chair sideways for position 2, the chair back creates a built-in visual and physical boundary between Tommy and Audrey **(Figure 6.5)**. Ms Zinn asks everyone to share their project with the buddy sitting next to them.

Now Louise is addressing two elements of A SECRET simultaneously: *relationship* and *environment*. Audrey and Tommy will be sharing crayons and glue, and Louise has created an environmental modification—a sort of low barrier—between the two children with the chair back. This helps Tommy stay within his boundaries, which is much better than being in Audrey's space. The two children now share the materials happily and giggle together while completing the task.

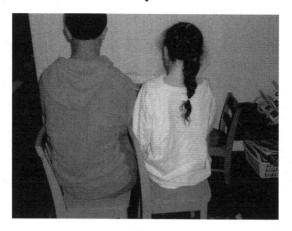

Figure 6.5. Chair Moves position 2 creates spatial boundaries between children by placing the backs of the chairs between them.

Great strides have been made with Tommy 20 minutes into the task, and for once, he hasn't gotten into trouble! "He probably only needs five or ten more minutes," thinks Louise. How can she add one more element to what has been accomplished today? Louise thinks about A SECRET and decides to modify the $T = Task$ element. What can she suggest about the writing task to help Tommy finish with a glow of success?

Louise can modify the paper Tommy is writing on by drawing lines with more defined borders or using two colors. In **Figure 6.6,** the dashes represent the middle of the "line" to help guide Tommy as he writes.

- - - - - I- - - - am- - - -like- - - -the- - - -animal.- - - - -

Figure 6.6. Modifying the task by substituting special writing paper.

This will help Tommy organize his written work on his paper. Tommy begins to tell the story of why he is like the donkey and president he cut out. He tells Miss Louise that he is going to write, "I am like a donkey because today I had long ears and listened to all the directions! And I am like the president today because I was the boss...the boss of my body! I did good, didn't I, Miss Louise?"

Additional Strategies to Use with Sensory Cravers

Table 6.8 summarizes additional useful strategies and activities to use with sensory-craving children.

Table 6.8. Strategies and Activities for Children with Sensory Craving

Sensory System	Strategies/Activities
Vestibular	*Start-and-Stop game.* The Start-and-Stop Game involves varying or interrupting movement. This game incorporates vestibular stimulation that starts and stops. Pictures of stop signs and stoplights can be shown to the children, or simple red, yellow, and green handmade squares can be used. First, the adult can flash a "signal," and the child must do whatever the color indicates: "green = go," "yellow = slow down," and "red = stop." Then the child can turn around and do it to the adult. (Children will get almost as much out of the activity by watching you do the right thing as they will from responding to the colors themselves. Also, this can be played peer-to-peer or in teams.) Use timers to stop and start. Incorporate jumping, rolling, climbing, and other types of vestibular input into the Start-and-Stop game in a varied fashion. Kickboxing, karate, and/or other martial arts provide purposeful, goal-directed movement combined with tactile, proprioceptive, and vestibular input.

Proprioceptive	Do goal-directed heavy-work activities prior to undertaking sitting tasks.
	Do joint compression and stretching activities paired with the vestibular input (eg, wheelbarrow-walking, body-sock play, or jumping on a trampoline while catching a weighted ball).
	Have the child wear compression garments under his clothes for small periods of time just before a time when he tends to get wound up.
	Have him make a stress ball out of balloons and sand that he can squeeze when needed.
Oral-Motor	Provide a balance of crunchy, chewy, and sucking oral-motor input.
Auditory	Use listening programs or music that provides lower sound frequencies for calming and sensorimotor skill development.
Tactile	Provide functional fidget tools.
	Introduce activities that involve deep-pressure input, such as massage, vibration, and brushing of the skin (with pressure).
Visual	Use visual cues to guide movements.
	Use motor movement charts, like *S'Cool Moves for Learning,* when transitioning from less structured gross-motor activities.
	Use motor charts placed outside the classroom prior to doing sit-down work.
Olfactory	Introduce calming scents, such as lavender, vanilla, or coconut.

Functional Fidget Tools

Functional fidget tools are available at different shops and Web sites and have been used by teachers and therapists in an attempt to help children focus while learning in the classroom. Functional fidget tools can be far more effective when used as a tool to help children attend and stay focused *simultaneous* to learning.

What Is a Functional Fidget Tool?

A functional fidget tool should have few sensory features, so the child doesn't become overloaded or distracted by the object. Rather, the child can finger it almost unconsciously while attending to a task. Fidget tools are small and fit easily into a child's hand(s). They're smooth, with no distracting features. They have few—if any—moving parts. Children often use functional fidget tools in the classroom, at the movies, during lunch in the cafeteria, or when entering into a new, worrisome situation.

Functional fidget tools are different than *commercial* fidget tools and/or sensory play objects and toys. The latter offer multiple forms of sensory input and can be distracting when a child needs to demonstrate performance-based concentration. Examples of everyday objects that can be used as functional fidget tools include paper clips, rubber bands, pen tops, smooth rocks, and pendants with engraved motivational sayings, such as "If you think you can or you think you can't, you're right." Be creative. There are endless options, most of which can be found around your house or classroom or purchased for practically nothing at a dollar store or thrift shop. As long as the fidget object doesn't take any thinking to play with, it may be worth trying to see if it enhances your child's attention level and ability to learn.

The purpose of using functional fidget tools is similar to that of chewing gum, but they are often more acceptable in classrooms because they won't be found stuck underneath a desk or on someone's shoes. The "perfect" functional fidget object for each child differs. You may need to try several options before you find just the right one.

To determine if the fidget tool is "just right," place a few functional fidget items on the child's desk when he is working on a cognitive or academic task. Observe whether the student chooses any objects over and over again and whether the object focuses the child or distracts him from completing tasks. **Table 6.9** offers guidelines when determining if the functional fidget tool is providing the type of sensory input required to enhance arousal and attention.

Table 6.9. Guidelines for Choosing Functional Fidget Tools

	Answer "Yes" or "No" to the Following Questions:	Yes	No
1.	Does the child attend better when holding or manipulating the functional fidget tool?		
2.	Does the child bring the fidget object with him to different settings?		
3.	Does the fidget object have only one primary sensory property?		
4.	Does the fidget object create an automatic response rather than produce a source of distraction?		
5.	Is the fidget object fairly ordinary and not desirable to every child in the classroom?		
6.	Can the fidget object be used in most situations (eg, in the classroom, at home, and in social environments)?		
7.	Is the fidget object easy to replace if lost?		

If the tool has 7 "yes" characteristics, it's an excellent fidget tool.

If the tool has 5-6 "yes" characteristics, it's a satisfactory fidget tool.

If the tool has 3-4 "yes" characteristics, it's a poor fidget tool.

If the tool has 1-2 "yes" characteristics, it's likely not to work.

Allow the child to use his or her chosen functional fidget tool for as long as needed to help reach a better arousal state for learning and task completion.

Using Chair Moves for Children
with Sensory Craving

Presenting options to allow the child to make frequent changes in position will bring tremendous relief to him in terms of his need for proprioceptive input during extended sitting activities. As the child moves the position of his chair during class or at home, a variety of different proprioceptive messages are sent to his brain. This is like a robust menu for the child's body and postpones the need to run around, touch things, fall out of his chair, and generally create chaos.

Five chair positions are incorporated into this program. Be creative and make up even more Chair Moves as you (or your child) think of them. These Chair Moves will only work if parents and teachers agree ahead of time that as long as the child is not disruptive, he or she can choose any Chair Moves on the list and change positions as desired. The child or—even better—the whole class can use Chair Moves throughout the day, depending on the activity the children are involved in. Remember how much better all the children did when a *purpose and goal* were paired with an activity and movement.

The most difficult job the sensory craver has when it comes to being able to complete classroom tasks is that he or she may be required to stay seated during task completion. These children often look for mischief, interrupt, and demonstrate behaviors that are not conducive to learning in class. Chair Moves is a program that shows therapists, teachers, and parents a variety of positions that allow a child to move by using his chair as a focal point during individual or group class sessions. The movement in the chair gives the child the ability and permission to move in a contained area and appears to enhance arousal states for learning. The positions are fun and easy to use in classrooms, at home, or during therapy sessions. As discussed in chapter 3 on emotional regulation, the five different positions of the chair can be laminated and placed on a small key ring for reference or taped to children's desks, binders, or folders. This will encourage a child with sensory-craving behaviors to remember to use Chair Moves for self-regulation. This strategy may also be useful with children who have sensory-based motor disorder, postural disorder, and/or sensory underresponsivity.

Chair Move 1—The first position of Chair Moves involves turning the chair around, so the back support faces the front **(Figure 6.7)**. The child straddles the chair. This is referred to as the "ride the pony" position and helps the child remember how to sit on the chair properly. It helps with arousal in that the child sits without back support and must use his own muscles to sit upright. Movement and proprioception are inherent to this position and are frequently noted as the child holds onto the top of the seat, perhaps pulling back slightly for some vestibular input. Activities such as cutting with scissors, coloring, gluing, and even having a snack may be more fun when children do not feel locked into a single, set position.

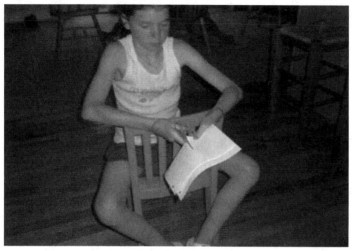

Figure 6.7. A child demonstrates Chair Moves position 1, with the seat back facing the front.

A child with a postural weakness can also benefit from using Chair Moves position 1 when using both hands together for self-help skills (such as buttoning and zipping). Having the back of the chair propped up against the child's chest as a gentle tactile cue provides reminders to use upright trunk strength while sitting. Activities such as eating, cutting, and using manipulative toys are made easier when the child has the postural support of the chair in the front, assisting him with holding his plate with the "helping" hand while using a fork or spoon in the dominant hand.

In Chair Moves positions 2 and 3, the child sits on the chair sideways **(Figure 6.8)**. Turning the chair toward either side allows for more movement when doing bilateral activities in the classroom or at home. Turning the chair toward the left side is position 2, and turning it toward the right side is position 3. The side-sit also gives the sensory craver a sense of freedom in space, yet provides a structured format for moving in the classroom while still attending well and focusing on what is going on around him or her.

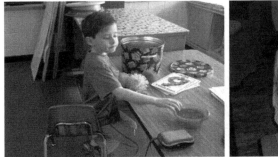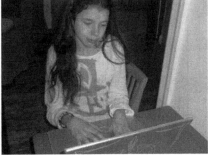

Figure 6.8. Chair Moves positions 2 and 3 involve turning the back of the chair to the side.

In Chair Moves position 4, the child kneels on the chair with one knee, with his other foot on the floor **(Figure 6.9)**. The child with sensory craving enjoys using this position, as it allows him to shift his weight and generate subtle vestibular input. This is a great position for listening and attending during story time and for reading, as sensory cravers often have difficulty remaining in seated positions and become distracted easily. This position is used less for fine-motor activities, because it is not a "stable" position.

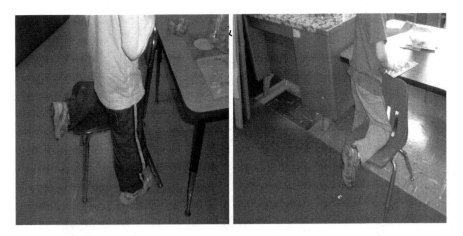

Figure 6.9. Chair Moves position 4 allows the child to bear weight on one knee during task completion.

In Chair Moves position 5, the child kneels on the chair with both legs, with the back of chair against the thighs **(Figure 6.10)**. This position enhances the ability to attend and can also provide a stable base while performing a writing activity or a two-handed fine-motor task. This alternative for children with sensory craving can have an organizing effect, because some small movements are permitted without being overly disruptive—like gently tapping the back of the chair, shifting the body weight from one knee to the other, or sitting back on the calves and then raising the body to a full kneeling position.

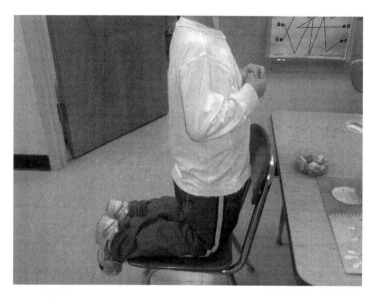

Figure 6.10. A child kneels on a chair in Chair Moves position 5 while performing a task in the classroom.

No Longer A SECRET

7

Sensory Discrimination Disorder

Sensory discrimination disorder is the second major pattern of SPD. Children with sensory discrimination disorder have difficulty differentiating between similar stimuli and deriving meaning from both internal and external sensory input in at least one or more sensory systems. For example, "cap" may sound the same as "cat," or a nickel may look and feel like a dime. Pushing softly may feel the same as pushing hard. A minor stomachache may feel extremely painful. Movement upward may be indistinguishable from movement downward. Thousands of subtle cues that most of us take for granted every day can be enigmatic and extremely confusing for kids whose senses can't sort out even these most basic descriptive messages.

What Is Sensory Discrimination Disorder?

It is common for a child to have excellent discrimination in one sensory domain, yet have difficulties with discrimination in other sensory domains. For example, a child may have excellent visual discrimination but poor auditory and/or tactile discrimination.

Note: In this book, we use the word "discrimination" to refer to the highest-level cognitive components of interpreting sensation. We realize other words can be used to refer to this high-level ability, such as *perception* or *detection*. *Discrimination,* in our context, refers to the higher-level executive function tasks of processing and interpreting sensory stimuli; this is a high-level task of not only comparing and contrasting stimuli but also interpreting or deriving meaning out of basic sensory stimuli that are detected.

Behaviors and Symptoms of
Sensory Discrimination Disorder

Children with sensory discrimination disorder have difficulty in one or more sensory systems. They have trouble distinguishing between the size, quality, shape, and texture of sounds, sights, and other sensory stimuli. Difficulty in differentiating qualitative and quantitative properties leads to confusion, misinterpretation, and problems in classifying elements of the environment, tasks, relationships, and other experiences that make these stimuli meaningful.

Children with sensory discrimination disorder have difficulty at the most basic level in determining what's the same and what's different about sensory stimuli, such as a written *b* versus *d* or discriminating the word "robe" from the word "rope."

Consider the principles involved in playing the game "Charades." A player challenges an opponent to try and guess what movie, book, or song is being acted out. On the basis of the cues presented, the opponent observes salient characteristics being acted out and tries to guess the word or phrase in question. The game opens many opportunities for discrimination mistakes among even the most traditionally developing players. But for kids with auditory discrimination disorder, the parameter "sounds like" would be extremely difficult for them to guess. Every day, each of us is barraged by thousands of sensory messages. For children with sensory discrimination disorder, life can truly be a guessing game.

The crucial aspect of understanding and recognizing sensory discrimination disorder is that it often masquerades as a behavioral problem. Here are some examples of how sensory discrimination disorder is mistakenly assumed to be a behavioral issue in each sensory system:

Sensory System	Behavior Mistaken as a Behavioral Issue
Tactile system	Is unable to dress quickly
Proprioceptive system	Has poor penmanship
Auditory system	Has difficulty following detailed directions or is slow to respond
Visual system	Reads slowly or poorly
Vestibular system	Is afraid of jumping short distances (is unable to judge distances above the ground)
Gustatory system (taste/texture)	Is a picky eater
Olfactory system (smell)	Refuses to go into certain restaurants
Interoceptive system	Is frequently in the nurse's office at school

Let's talk about discrimination as it pertains to each sensory domain.

Touch or tactile domain.—Discrimination in this domain refers to sensing touch and localizing where the input occurred. It includes knowing what you have touched without seeing it (called *stereognosis*). If a child has a tactile discrimination disorder, he will typically try to compensate by using his vision. For example, a child may not feel the pencil well enough to write letters or numbers clearly. The child may squint, hold the pencil incorrectly, or bend his head close to the pencil to try to compensate. (See **Table 7.1.**)

Table 7.1 Symptoms of Tactile Discrimination Disorder

Symptoms of Tactile Discrimination Disorder	
	Has difficulty buttoning and finding the buttons and button holes without guiding the fingers with the eyes
	Has difficulty identifying an object when it is only touched and not seen (as in reaching inside one's desk for a pencil and finding it by using touch only)
	Has difficulty knowing where a scratch or bruise is on one's body
	Has difficulty using similar objects (may think a paper clip is a safety pin according to touch alone)
	Has difficulty recognizing objects on the basis of differentiating features, such as shape, texture, and size, especially if only part of the object can be seen—for example, if a toothbrush is partly covered by a washcloth, the child may not recognize it as a whole toothbrush, thinking it is a stick instead
	Has difficulty differentiating temperatures—this can present safety concerns for children with sensory discrimination disorder

Proprioceptive domain.—This sense is responsible for knowing "just the right amount" of tension or force required when responding to various environmental demands. Carrying a juice box while walking down stairs requires a child to use "just the right amount" of force and tension, or else he may squeeze the box too hard and spurt juice all over the stairs.

Proprioceptive discrimination disorder occurs when there is difficulty grading the tension needed for a task—in other words, the force from one's muscles does not match the task demands. Children who are developing typically learn very quickly how much force and muscle tension they should use in any given situation through trial and error. Objects become associated with distinguishing characteristics. Seeing a specific object in the environment automatically and often unconsciously prepares the child's system to set up and use the right amount of force required.

A child with sensory discrimination disorder may at first seem like a child who is underresponsive or has postural disorder, and of course both disorders are often seen simultaneously. For example, is it sensory underresponsivity or sensory discrimination disorder that causes a child to slouch in the chair, have a hard time following his teacher's voice in a noisy classroom, or use so little pressure when writing that the letters are barely visible? Careful observation can help differentiate whether the sensory input is being interpreted correctly and/or whether the child is not regulating his responses to sensory stimuli. Symptoms of a discrimination disorder in the proprioceptive sensory system are described in **Table 7.2.**

Table 7.2. Symptoms of Proprioceptive Discrimination Disorder

Symptoms of Proprioceptive Discrimination Disorder	Has difficulty using the correct amount of pressure with glue sticks, markers, pencils, paper clips, hole punchers, and staplers
	Has difficulty judging and using the correct amount of pressure and force during motor tasks like throwing a ball, hitting a target, kicking a ball, and opening and closing doors
	Has difficulty judging a safe amount of force to use when participating in full-body contact sports, such as wrestling, kickboxing, or martial arts (or even playing "tag!")
	Is unable to judge how much force and tension to use while pedaling uphill or downhill
	Has difficulties dressing (eg, using the correct amount of force to put one's arms into the sleeve holes; pulling up one's socks with the toe section in front without having an awareness of how hard to pull to get the sock on; putting fingers into gloves using the correct amount force when placing the fingers into the finger holes)
	Has difficulty cutting through foods without loudly scraping the plate
	Has difficulty feeling how much effort to use while typing or playing a musical instrument
	Older girls may have difficulty judging how much force is needed to apply the correct amount of lipstick, mascara, or blush

Lily's Story

Lily is an 8-year-old girl with proprioceptive and tactile discrimination disorders. In many ways, she is successful. She is smart, has lots of friends, and does well in groups of kids. Her mother worries about her because she is always getting hurt and breaking things.

Lily runs up to her mother's car and flings open the car door; as it swings back against the car, the hinges practically rip out. She pulls the door shut by using so much force that the whole car shakes.

Lily has been playing at her friend's house. Her shoes are on the wrong feet, and her laces are open. Her jacket is not buttoned correctly, so one side is longer than the other. Lily's mother sees that Lily's hand is bleeding. "Lily, are you okay? What happened to your hand?" asks her mom.

Lily looks down at her hand and shrugs. "I think the cat scratched me, but I'm not sure," she answers.

"Well be sure to wash it off when you get home," replies her mother.

Lily doesn't really know where her body is in relation to the everyday objects around her. She doesn't discriminate pain very well (people are always praising her for being brave, but she doesn't even notice cuts, bruises, or scrapes).

Visual domain.—A child with poor visual discrimination has trouble distinguishing characteristics of similar objects, emotional expressions, and written symbols. Poor visual discrimination skills often lead to a child experiencing a number of academic and learning issues. These can include letter and number reversals, poor mapping skills and inadequate abilities in finding routes (such as from home to school), difficulty finding key words or objects in pictures, trouble trying to find differences in pictures that look similar, difficulty with reading at the proper grade level, and challenges in finding and distinguishing small objects on the floor, in a drawer, or inside a backpack.

A child with visual discrimination disorder may end up trying to figure out what is happening by staring at other children's work. He or she may be mislabeled as a cheater or being "slow." Often not recognized but most problematic is the likelihood that children with visual discrimination difficulties will have problems reading the facial expressions of teachers, parents, or peers. Many interpersonal and social problems arise when the child misreads visual cues or is misunderstood (eg, "Wipe that smirk off your face, young man. Do you want to go to the principal's office?") (See **Table 7.3.**)

Table 7.3. Symptoms of Poor Visual Discrimination

Symptoms of Visual Discrimination Disorder	Has difficulty recognizing symbols on traffic signs
	Has difficulty lining up number columns on paper
	Has difficulty choosing a key from a key ring for a specific lock
	Has difficulty telling time by judging the spatial orientation of numbers on the face of a clock
	Has difficulty scanning a page and finding key words in text
	Has difficulty parking and judging distances between a car and a curb, a fire hydrant, or a pedestrian
	Has difficulty changing lanes and merging into oncoming traffic while driving

Auditory domain.—Children with auditory discrimination disorder often seem as if they're not listening or comprehending what is said. Our environment is filled with constant and diverse auditory input, such as dogs barking, sirens blaring, phones ringing, vacuum cleaners humming, and classmates (or office mates) chatting. Children with auditory discrimination problems often have difficulty identifying one sound (eg, Mom calling their name) from a cacophony of background sounds, which is technically called an *auditory figure-ground* difficulty. Auditory figure-ground problems have a profound effect on young children who are required to attend, listen to a teacher's directions, and block out distracting noises.

There are potentially many more components to an auditory discrimination disorder, including difficulty sequencing sounds (for instance, saying "aminal" instead of "animal"). If the disorder goes unrecognized for too long, the child may be labeled as having a speech impediment, behavioral issues, or attention-deficit disorder.

Note that a central auditory processing disorder is a subset of auditory discrimination disorder, a very specific type of disorder. Central auditory processing disorder interferes with the processing of auditory stimuli and attaching meaning in context to what is being heard. Many children benefit from structured programs designed for that purpose. Audiologists who specialize in central auditory processing disorder use filters that are embedded into the ear to assist children with hearing sounds accurately.[42]

In the area of visual and auditory discrimination disorders, there are dozens of existing treatments, such as the Lindamood-Bell Program, the Wilson Reading Program, and many others. In the area of audition, there are several good programs on the market that involve listening to modulated classical music, such as Integrated Listening Systems. The child listens to the music through headphones that have a built-in vibration mechanism to provide bone conduction and stimulate the vestibular system.

Suzanne's Story

"How many times do I have to call your name?" yells Suzanne's mother. Suzanne is in her room, looking at *Teen Vogue*. In the background are the competing sounds of the dog barking, the dishwasher swishing, her siblings fighting, her dad singing in the shower, her CD playing, and—somewhere deep within her realm of consciousness—her mom calling for her to come down to the kitchen. Because Suzanne has an auditory discrimination disorder, she has trouble picking out one background sound from all the sounds around her.

Suzanne isn't ignoring her mother or being disrespectful. She processes her mom's voice as being background noise—just another sound in her busy house. Her mom is getting angry.

"Suzanne, if you don't get down here in one minute, you are going to have to wash all the dishes," her mother yells up the stairs. "You are so lazy! That's it—I've had it with you."

Finally, as her mom's voice pitch rises to an unusually high level, Suzanne becomes aware that she's hearing something out of the ordinary in her environment. She comes out of her room to see what's going on. She's met with her mom's exasperation.

"Why do I have to call you over and over? Why are ignoring me? We've talked about your laziness many times. Do you think I'm your slave? That's it, young lady. You can't go to Leslie's party tonight. And if you don't change your attitude...well, let's just say you're going to regret it."

Feeling she's been unjustly blamed, Suzanne bursts into tears, runs into her room, and slams the door, making her seem even less cooperative.

There is so much misunderstanding in this vignette. This is obviously an often-repeated scenario in Suzanne's house. If parents and teachers do not know that a child has an auditory processing problem, they may expect the child to hear and participate, when in actuality, the child is unable to discern the words being said. The tragedy of Suzanne's story is that she herself may soon come to believe that she is "lazy or dumb." A lack of self-esteem may preclude her from doing well at school and, eventually, from rising to meet other challenges or responsibilities later in life. Undiagnosed auditory processing problems can have huge consequences for children—for life. One youngster said recently, "Everyone thinks I'm bad—I guess I may as well be bad, instead of trying so hard to do things right." (See **Table 7.4.**)

Table 7.4. Symptoms of Auditory Discrimination Disorder

Symptoms of Auditory Discrimination Disorder	
	Has difficulty recognizing the differences between sounds (eg, "hard" vs "heart"; "bag" vs "back" vs "bat")
	Has difficulty in distinguishing which direction a sound is coming from (localizing sounds)
	Has poor listening skills, which affects descriptive language vocabulary and the ability to follow directions
	Talks too loudly or too softly
	Has poor articulation of certain words (a child tends to be unable to say what he or she cannot hear)
	Has difficulty rhyming words (this is an early sign that a child should be tested for auditory processing disorder)
	Experiences confusion with words that sound alike and often misuses and/or substitutes words in sentences
	Has trouble differentiating emotions related to voices (eg, angry voices vs happy voices)
	Experiences confusion and acts like he or she is "in a fog" for much of the day

> *You only need two of the following three sensory systems to balance:*
>
> *1. Visual*
>
> *2. Vestibular*
>
> *3. Proprioceptive*
>
> *If a child has balance problems, it is critical to determine which of the two senses is affected so that intervention can be targeted to the right sensory system.*

Vestibular domain.—For kids to move and balance, adequate sensory messages need to arrive from the vestibular, visual, and/or proprioceptive systems. The vestibular system helps determine where our head is in space, relative to gravity. If a child has difficulty with vestibular discrimination, he may not feel when he is starting to fall and will not be able to catch himself before he gets hurt. If his visual and proprioceptive systems are the two systems keeping him balanced, things may work well until either one is disabled (eg, in a birthday party game of "pin the tail on the donkey," in which a child may not be able to function when blindfolded). If the proprioceptive system is impaired, a child will have difficulty walking on an uneven surface or up and down stairs with his vision occluded. This discussion is admittedly rather technical, but it has implications for what therapists choose to target in treatment. It takes an advanced therapist to be able to sort out what is causing a child's balance problems, but parents and teachers can benefit by asking for an evaluation of the causes of balance difficulties if their child experiences this problem. (See **Table 7.5.**)

Table 7.5. Symptoms of Vestibular Discrimination Disorder

Symptoms of Vestibular Discrimination Disorder	Has a poor awareness of where and when the body is moving in space
	Has difficulty changing directions when moving (eg, rolling, moving onto the hands and knees, getting up onto the knees, then standing, as you might see in any football or soccer game)
	Has difficulty moving at all when the eyes are closed (although this seems rather abstract, a child with this difficulty is going to have trouble with team sports and any physical activity—he will not be able to keep up with his friends at the playground or swimming pool or at a sports field)
	Knows that he is falling but can't tell which way

Olfactory and gustatory domains.—In chapter 6, we described the significance of taste and smell for altering arousal states in children with sensory underresponsiveness. Children with sensory discrimination disorder sometimes, but not always, have sensory underresponsiveness in addition to sensory discrimination disorder. In fact, a child with smell and taste sensory discrimination disorder may not be able to tell the differences between "calming" or "alerting" types of smells and foods, in which case it is difficult to use smell as an arousal stimulus for sensory underresponsiveness. It can also work in reverse; if a child has sensory underresponsiveness in the olfactory system, his or her discrimination in that system is almost guaranteed to be poor. If the sensory underresponsiveness is alleviated, sometimes children with sensory discrimination disorders in smell and taste start to discriminate much better. This can lead to improved eating and socially appropriate participation in restaurant experiences and other situations where odors can be an issue. (See **Table 7.6.**)

Table 7.6. Symptoms of Olfactory/Gustatory Discrimination Disorder

Symptoms of Olfactory/Gustatory Discrimination Disorder	
	Has difficulty distinguishing sweet, salty, bitter, and spicy foods
	Is a picky eater; a child may base "liking" foods on the visual presentation if he has difficulty smelling or tasting food
	Displays an unwillingness to try food he hasn't tasted before
	Does not like restaurants unless the food is predictable (eg, McDonald's)
	Refuses to enter a restaurant or sit at a certain table because of the way it "smells"
	Complains about hugging "Aunt Mary" because of the way she smells
	Refuses to use a towel that has been in the dryer with a particular type of dryer sheet
	Refuses to use public bathrooms because of the smell

Sensory Discrimination Disorder

Interoceptive domain.—When a child with an interoceptive discrimination disorder tries to interpret sensory messages from her internal organs, she may have a general sense of malaise but be unable to pinpoint the problem. In this domain, sensory discrimination disorder affects the ability to decipher messages from interoceptors. Children feel confused by sensory messages and are unable to assess their internal environment correctly.

This disorder sets children up to be viewed as a "child who cries wolf." The child may exhibit frequent, nonspecific complaints about what and where the pain and discomfort are, which ultimately causes the adults around her to not take her feedback seriously. (See **Table 7.7.**)

Table 7.7. Symptoms of Interoceptive Discrimination Disorder

Symptoms of Interoceptive Discrimination Disorder	
	Has somatic complaints, which are often vague and difficult to pinpoint—"My stomach feels weird" might mean anything from having a mild stomachache to being ready to throw up
	Is unaware of feeling of hunger, thirst, or a sensation of being satiated or full
	Ends up in the nurse's office at school more frequently than being in the classroom; has frequent school absences
	May confuse emotional states with sensations from her organs—"I am angry and depressed" may really be a reflection of sensations from inside her body

Principles of Intervention for Sensory Discrimination Disorder

The following discussion presents the key principles of intervention for children who have sensory discrimination disorder.

Principle 1. Assist children in being aware of properties of people, objects, and other things.

Help children begin to appreciate the unique sensory qualities of objects to be able to differentiate one from another. Through awareness of these qualities, the meaning of stimuli becomes apparent. We derive pleasure from the deeper appreciation of qualities of objects, events, and people in our world. Smelling a flower, tasting a ripe pear, feeling the hug of a loved one, reading a great poem, listening to Mozart…all of these experiences require discrimination, meaning the ability to interpret sensory stimuli. Without this ability, we feel less joy. Understanding the meaning of sensory stimulation infuses our lives with a deeper quality of richness.

Principle 2. Infuse rich descriptions of sensorimotor play into activities you do together.

When playing with your child, try to make note of as many descriptive aspects as possible. For example, you could address the properties of objects you're playing with, including size, shape, quantity, quality, and texture. If your child is older and can handle more challenging conversations, talk about the different ways things can be classified (eg, "Let's find all the round items in this room").

Play the "find it" game while driving. "Let's find everything we pass that is blue—first it's my turn, and then it's your turn," you might say. Note that the activity will generally work much better if you play, too. Alternate with your child in choosing questions. "Let's see if we can find every place that serves food," he says. And you say, "Let's see if we can find every place that costs money." And so on. Categorizing their surroundings helps kids discern what's the same versus what is different—which is a stepping stone to discrimination.

Principle 3. Communication is our most important human attribute.

Descriptors are immensely important in communication. For example, take the statement, "I feel bad." We learn so much more if a descriptor is provided, such as "I feel bad because I'm so tired," or "I feel bad because my muscles are sore from lifting weights," or "I feel bad because my stomach hurts." Use descriptors in normal conversation to cue your child on an everyday basis.

Principle 4. Work on visualization.

Visualization is essential to reading, writing, and many other tasks. Before you can write a letter, you have to hold it in your mind. Thus, games like a *hiding game,* in which you put something inside of a box or pillowcase and have your child guess what it is, are a great way to encourage him or her to visualize and differentiate objects. Write large numbers and letters in the air before putting them down on paper. Have your child use words to describe what he sees (visualize) before writing the letters down (eg, visualize whether the letter is round or has lines, and whether there are up-and-down lines or diagonal lines). Have the child make his body into letters, shapes, and numbers. Play a game like "I Spy," but have it be "I'm thinking of…" and you guess details, while the child says "yes" or "no" to each question related to what he or she is visualizing.

Principle 5. Measure and weigh things around you.

Weighing and measuring things is not only helpful for discrimination—it also forms the foundation for learning mathematics. These are easy concepts for children to master because they are so concrete. Travel through your child's world with a soft measuring tape or a small kitchen scale. Baking and planting are great activities that the whole family can do to practice weighing and measuring. Really, in a child's world, almost everything can be weighed or measured.

> ## Principle 6. Play games that provide information about "same" and "different."

While standing in line at the grocery store, discuss edible versus nonedible items, sweet-smelling and sour-smelling items, big versus small items, red versus blue items, etcetera. Play a similar game while driving. The more opportunities your child has to appreciate the specific qualities around him or her, the more quickly discrimination abilities are likely to advance. Even making homemade play dough by adding salt, pepper, garlic, lemon, and different-smelling extracts helps your child experience an array of smells.

> ## Principle 7. Practice activities that require your child to use unusual positions and sustain balance.

Do activities or play games in which your child changes his body position (such as "Simon Says" or "Twister"). Cue your child to describe how he changed his body position, such as, "I moved my leg to the side," or "I moved my hand up to the red circle." Make sure you help your child describe his feelings about positions that are hard for him to move into during the activity. This will help enhance his body sense and self-awareness.

A SECRET for Sensory Discrimination Disorder

Let's use A SECRET framework to address the multiple challenges that arise for children with sensory discrimination disorder.

You can help your child by slowly exposing him to things that are difficult, without a sense of stress or pressure. For example, if it's tough for him to attend to sounds with competing background auditory stimuli, do not remove all the noise from his environment all the time. Instead, gradually introduce the level and differentiation of sound in his environment. There are many activities to assist children with discrimination disorder. **Table 7.8** suggests strategies for this purpose.

Table 7.8. A SECRET for Sensory Discrimination Disorder

Element from A SECRET	Activity	Purpose
Attention	*Snap-and-Clap Game.* Read a story that contains names of animals and action words. Use a varied tone, and don't show any pictures of the words being read. The child listens and responds to the specific words in the story by snapping or clapping to specific cues, such as, "Every time I say 'the rabbit,' you clap." "Every time I say the word 'he,' you snap."	Helps with auditory figure-ground discrimination, which increases attention; is good practice in attending to and filtering out irrelevant background sounds, shapes, and forms both with and without visual cues.
Sensation	Activities like "Twister" and "Hokey Pokey" involve movement related to the location of specific body parts. These are just two of many such activities. Put something into the child's hand that he cannot see. In this game, he feels it without using visual cues and guesses what object he is holding. The goal is for the child to match objects to identical shapes or forms by feeling its three-dimensional properties first. When he has mastered this, have him match what he feels to a photo of the object.	Improves a child's awareness of the location of his body and body parts and the movement of his body through space.

Emotional Regulation	The child can act in a leadership role while playing games like "Charades" or "Taboo." The child gets an opportunity to offer clues about objects. This game requires the child to use descriptors to give clues to other children, who guess what the objects are. Being a leader and cueing other children take the pressure off the child and, at the same time, cast him as a leader who has self-control.	Encourages the child to be a leader, emphasizing his ability to exercise self-control and cue other children to use descriptors, adjectives, and other words to categorize and differentiate objects from one another.
Culture	Change the culture of the types of games typically played by your family and your child by incorporating more games that use visual cues as reminders. The "Find and Feel, Show It on the Wheel" activity (Activity 7A, directions follow) can help children with discrimination disorders become better at providing clues to describe objects to others.	Changes the culture of game-playing by mixing up the sequence of how games are played, by asking the child to use descriptors about quantity and quality *prior to playing games.*
Relationship	Play "Charades," bake, garden, hike, walk, measure, weigh, and explore with your child. Focus on exploring your relationship with your child, and discover new qualities of the world around you.	Share with your child; communication is one of the most important attributes that makes us human. Your child's best role model is you!

Environment	Help your child organize his environment in a fun way. Use color, shape, size, weight, and a variety of other elements to enhance sensory discrimination. This will help your child learn to differentiate similarities and differences in objects. You might put blue stickers on everything that starts with *B* or red stickers on everything used for homework.	Labeling the environment and categorizing things in his surroundings helps your child learn to discriminate.
Task	Offer a choice of materials for the child to complete a particular task. For example, ask, "Do you want light tracing paper or construction paper to cut out a silhouette of your body? Do you want loop scissors or regular scissors to cut out the valentine hearts? Do you want green putty or red putty to make the pots for your mom? Do you want markers or crayons to color the large chart? Constantly asking questions that differentiate qualities of A vs B will reinforce the discriminative characteristics of the world around the child.	Offering the child options to help with task success requires the child to discriminate between heavy vs light, hard vs soft, and other properties.

How-To Activities

In this section, we provide easy "how-to" directions for recommended activities for children with sensory discrimination disorder. These suggestions are cost-effective and fun to use with one or more children. Games are perfect for playing on the weekends with siblings or when your child has a playdate.

Activity 7A. Find It, Feel It, Show It on the Wheel

How to make the activity elements:

1. To start, cut a large circle out of white poster paper. On the circle, use a ruler to divide the circle up into eight sections **(Figure 7.1)**.

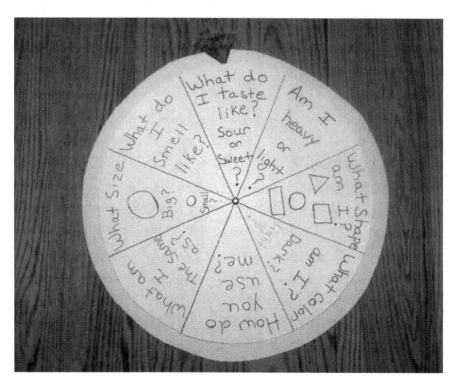

Figure 7.1. A circle with eight sections marked off for the game "Find It, Feel It, Show It on the Wheel."

Put specific descriptors on each section, such as size (big, small), shape (round, square), smell, color (dark, bright), weight (heavy, light), and taste (sweet, sour, salty). You can add other descriptors to the circle and/or change them around.

2. The wheel is fastened to cardboard or a heavy piece of paper with a small brad (fastener) that allows it to spin.

3. Place a black arrow on the border of the paper to indicate the specific section of the circle that has been selected.

How to play the game:

Create a list of objects and/or items that meet the criteria of the descriptors. Choose the order in which the game will be played. The first child (Child A) spins the descriptor wheel. Once the wheel stops spinning, it will land on a section of the wheel. Child B must choose two items that fit the descriptors. Hopefully, each child does not run out of ideas for objects. The items that they guess must be on the list that you created. If they're having trouble coming up with guesses, are there clues to help them get on the right track? Each correct guess gets one point. The first child to get 10 points can win a small prize from, say, a tiny treasure chest.

Activity 7B. Say It, Play It with Clay

This is a spinoff of Activity 7A that has been incredibly successful with children with discrimination disorders! In this activity, Child A chooses an object and writes it down. Then, Child A creates the object out of clay or play dough.

Child B looks at the clay model and, on the basis of its distinguishing features, tries to guess what the object is. Child B must use descriptive words that relate to his idea of what the object is. If you were observing this game, it might sound like this:

"I think you made a bunny because of the long, floppy ears, the little, round, puffy tail, and the almond-shaped eyes. You used play dough that's white, which bunnies often are."

It's like playing "Charades," but it involves sculpting the object rather than acting it out. This helps Child A incorporate the distinguishing characteristics of the object, while Child B has to visualize and put together all the properties to form the percept of the object **(Figure 7.2)**.

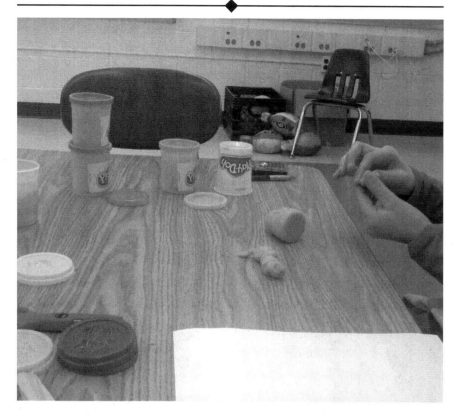

Figure 7.2. Use descriptors to make objects out of clay or play dough.

Activity 7C. What's in Your Hand?

This is a fun and easy activity to put together for children on any rainy day. Collect a bunch of small objects from your kitchen that are familiar to your child. If you are using unfamiliar objects, like a spool of thread, get two of the same—one for your child to feel and the other for your child to point to after feeling the object in his hand.

For familiar objects, ask your child descriptive questions, such as, "What shape are you feeling—is it big or small, sharp or dull," etcetera. For unfamiliar items, set the object pairs on the table and ask the child to point to the same item as the one he has in his hand. It is easy to create tactile discrimination activities that challenge the child to feel different textures, sizes, and shapes under a table **(Figure 7.3)**.

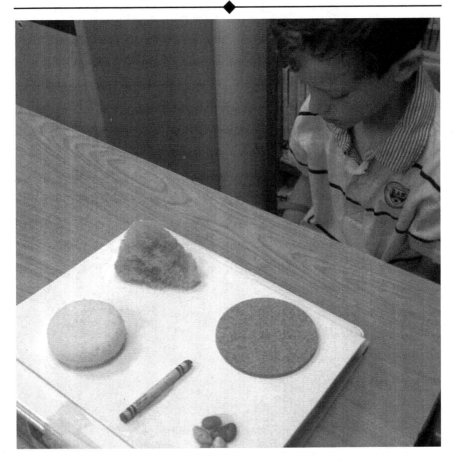

Figure 7.3. Some sample items used to play the
"What's in Your Hand?" game.

Activity 7D. What Do You Smell?

This activity involves using strongly scented or flavored extracts (like vanilla, peppermint, and almond). Cover the labels on the bottles of extract. Use index cards to draw a picture of what the extract is made out of (ie, draw an apple for "apple extract"). The child then smells the extract and tries to guess the flavor. The index cards placed in front of the child provide visual cues.

A small drop of flavor can be tasted if the child needs or wants additional hints regarding the extracts. This way, the child can use his senses of both smell and taste **(Figure 7.4)**.

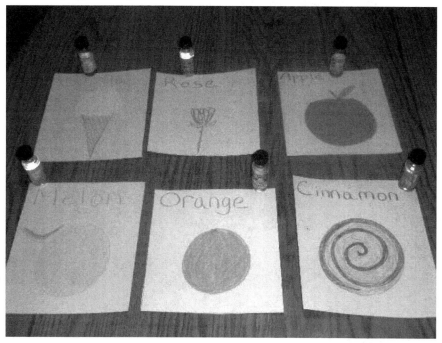

Figure 7.4. A depiction of how to play the "What Do You Smell?" game, involving scented extracts and visual aids. Visual aids created by K. A. Lawson.

Additional Activities for Sensory Discrimination Disorder

Table 7.9. Activities for Sensory Discrimination Disorder

Sensory System	Activities to Enhance Discrimination
Visual	Crossword puzzles Word searches Boggle or Scrabble "What's missing in the picture?" Weighted balls, beanbags, and bowling with targets
Auditory	Acting-out/role-playing games Rhyming games Hullabaloo Sound Bingo Sound Lotto Mad Libs
Proprioceptive	Operation "Don't Break the Ice" Jenga Jacks Mancala Balloon painting Blowing activities (for internal proprioception) Whack-a-Mole Mousetrap

Tactile	Textured dominoes (Tactominoes)
	Ned's Head
	Tracing
	Wikki Stix
	Color Wonder
	Invisible-inkpad games
Vestibular	Twister
	Playground equipment
	Teeter-totters
	Slides
	Swings
Taste/Smell	Scented markers or stickers

8

Sensory-based Motor Disorder—Postural Disorder

The third category of SPD, sensory-based motor disorder, includes two subtypes: postural disorder and dyspraxia. Sensory-based motor disorder is basically a motor disorder with an underlying sensory dysfunction. Sensory-based motor disorder is different than a modulation disorder because the children who manifest sensory-based motor disorder do not have problems regulating their responses to sensory stimulation. They are much less likely to have meltdowns or "zone out" from sensory input than are children with modulation disorders, although some sensory underresponsiveness is common.

Those with postural disorder have a lack of core strength and poor endurance for motor activities and, in particular, have difficultly *stabilizing* their bodies both when holding still and during movement. Stabilizing means contracting the muscles in the core (trunk), so that if someone were to push against you, you could remain *stable* and not fall or move.

Children with postural disorder have poor core strength and thus have difficulty with executing movements, due to weak muscles and poor awareness of body sensations—particularly in the tactile and proprioceptive domains. Children with dyspraxia (see chapter 9) also have a sensory-based motor disorder. They do not have weak core muscles but instead have trouble coming up with ideas for motor actions, planning, and sequencing the movements needed for an action and/or executing precise movement patterns.

To help visualize what postural disorder looks like, watch what happens to people at airports when they are required to get onto a moving walkway. Some people step right on and move quickly to the left side of the walkway, rolling their luggage behind them. Others appear to be very uncomfortable when walking on a moving surface with luggage. People who may have postural disorder remain on the right side of the walkway, holding on for dear life and making no attempt to walk on the moving surface. This is probably related to the discomfort they feel in moving their bodies simultaneously with being physically moved by an outside force. A fear of falling is often caused by the inability to stabilize the body during movement. Both children and adults with postural disorder will remain on the right side of the walkway, holding on tightly and letting others pass them by. (Of course, there are other reasons people ride on the right side too, such as being exhausted from traveling, wheeling heavy loads, or having vestibular problems, like experiencing dizziness on a moving sidewalk.)

What Is Postural Disorder?

Postural control refers to the ability to manage the movements of the muscles and joints. Children who receive accurate sensory input from their tactile, vestibular, and proprioceptive systems can climb up and down a tree knowing (but not necessarily being consciously aware of) where their hands and feet are while they're moving around. The "knowing" occurs because they are receiving accurate sensory feedback from their muscles, joints, and tendons; in other words, they are processing feedback from their proprioceptive systems. Proprioception provides body awareness and an internal map of where your body is in space. Walking or running on uneven surfaces, jumping off curbs, skipping, roller-skating, skiing, and lots of other active movements are fun and easy when you have postural control and intact proprioception.

In community settings, a child with postural control uses escalators without thinking about it, enjoys elevator rides, and can negotiate an active, moving sidewalk. Outdoor activities, such as helping her parents with the gardening and making a patio, are fun. The child knows where her body is in space through proprioception and can move comfortably and manipulate objects to complete tasks. A child with postural control has endurance and strength and enjoys the feelings of stretching and curling up her body. A good hike with her family in the mountains or on the seashore is fun for a child with postural control.

Postural disorder impedes many simple, everyday activities. A child with postural disorder can feel panic even during potty training, because she has difficulty stabilizing her body on the toilet seat. One youngster told me he thought he might fall in and get flushed away because his body was so wobbly. The daunting sight of the toilet rising up off the floor can produce anxiety and *somatic discomfort* (meaning "discomfort in your body"). If you have postural disorder, the toilet can be viewed as a dangerous place to sit; thus, a child tries to tighten all his muscles so he doesn't fall. This obviously interferes with the sensation of "letting go" needed to master bowel and bladder control.

Behaviors and Symptoms in Postural Disorder

With good postural abilities, children can push, pull, carry heavy objects, climb oddly shaped structures, and resist an unexpected force. For example, if another child accidently bumps into him, the child will not fall over. Children with postural challenges have trouble with all these actions. For example, instead of resisting the pull in tug-of-war, they tend to fall toward the direction of the opponents' pull. Children with postural disorder substitute *compensatory strategies* (attempts to counteract the force that puts their body into abnormal positions) to help stabilize body parts during motor tasks. One classic position every parent with a child in occupational therapy hears about is "W sitting," in which the child sits on the floor with his knees almost touching and his hips turned in, with his feet splayed wide apart behind his body to provide a wide base of support as he attempts to sit **(Figure 8.1)**.

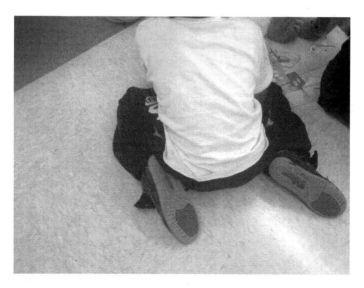

Figure 8.1. The "W" sitting position.

An example of this can be seen as Danny sits on his chair in the classroom during "quiet time." During "quiet time," Danny and his classmates are required to work independently and complete a packet of math work. Danny sits on one leg and leans his weight on his hands. When he's done thinking about a math problem, he picks up his pencil with one hand, but he doesn't hold down the paper with his other hand because he's resting his head on it. Sometimes the pencil is in his right hand, and sometimes it's in his left. Since he is not holding the math sheet down, it turns as he writes on it and gets positioned at an odd angle. Now, on top of his other issues, he has to deal with a visually distorted perception of the math problems, which further delays completion of the math packet.

Miss Craig, Danny's teacher, sees the difficulty he is having while working at his desk. She offers Danny the option of working at a "standing desk" while completing his work **(Figure 8.2)**. However, Danny has weak core muscles and poor strength and endurance and would rather stay seated in his chair, slumped over, completing his math work late.

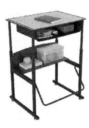

Figure 8.2. A "standing desk" (this one is from *www.schoolsin.com*).

At home, Danny chooses to watch TV, play on his computer, and be a passive bystander, watching his brother and his friends compete with each other on the Wii. Danny never plays on the Wii; he says, "It's too tiring and not fun at all!" The Wii requires postural control, which Danny does not have.

Barry's Story

Barry, a second-grader, dreads his next class—art. He hates it even more because everyone else loves it. Touching the art materials is not an issue for him like it would be for an overresponsive child, and he has no problems sequencing the steps to make the cool things that Miss Nelson shows them how to do. But Barry has a significant postural disorder, and the thought of sitting up on the high stool with nothing to put his back against is exhausting.

No Longer A SECRET

He knows that today when he arrives, he faces 45 minutes of art, with all the children laughing and talking, making different projects for Mother's Day. He grimaces, thinking about reaching across the table to share crayons, shifting his weight from side to side to get materials and see others' projects. But most of all, he is resentful that he will have to get up and down off the stool multiple times.

Halfway through art class, Barry knows he will not be able to finish his project unless he does something radical. He slips down onto the floor with his supplies and lies down to complete his project. He knows that if Miss Nelson sees him, she may send him to the principal's office—and he waits apprehensively. Finally, Miss Nelson does see him and says, "Barry—not again! How many times do I have to tell you not to lie down on the floor? Now sit up." Barry sighs and sits up in a "W position." Barry knows from experience that this is the most stable position in which to sit, although he prefers lying down on the floor. When sitting, Barry still bends his head as close to the floor as possible to work on his project.

Barry already knows he is *different;* in fact, all the kids keep telling him that, and now he can't even finish his Mother's Day project on time. *"I'm just a stupid mess,"* he thinks, *"and now I'll never get my Mother's Day project done."* Ironically, Barry is one of the most intelligent children in class.

Symptoms of Postural Disorder

If a child has postural disorder, part of his discomfort in moving comfortably around his environment is related to an imbalance in the strength of his muscle groups. He does not feel stable because muscles that usually fire together— such as the front and back of your leg (the quadriceps and hamstrings)— are not firing equally, contributing to what therapists call "poor muscle *co-contraction.*" In other words, either the front of your leg or the back of your leg (or your arm or trunk or neck) is stronger; therefore, the muscle contractions are unequal. As a result of *poor co-contraction*, a child ends up being pulled into the direction of the stronger muscle group. A series of related motor issues are noted with poor co-contraction, including problems in shifting weight and rotating the trunk. Without rotating, balance is compromised and many problems can ensue, such as not being able to resist a fall.

The combinations of issues noted in postural disorder stability interfere not only with balance, but also with the ability to sustain an upright position.

Thus, children may fall frequently. This is known as *instability* (or *postural instability*) because the children are not *stable*—meaning they cannot resist pressure against their bodies without falling.

Children with postural disorder who have to ride the school bus have a particularly difficult time. If the driver hits the brakes unexpectedly, they will likely fall to the ground, as they are unable to maintain their posture against a force pushing forward. These children are usually scared to death of falling, but everyone attributes their reluctance to ride the bus to a phobia or to an unreasonable fear of riding the bus. These children know their balance reactions are "not the greatest," and although they can't state it in these terms, the problem is that because of their lack of core strength, they can't support their bodies against any outside force.

Behaviors exhibited in a child with postural disorder appear primarily in the following sensory domains: vestibular, proprioceptive, tactile, and two motor areas: bilateral coordination (doing actions with both sides of the body at the same time) and the ocular-motor area (the coordinated use of the eyes during motor tasks). **Table 8.1** details the primary areas of difficulty for children with postural disorder.

Table 8.1. Areas of Difficulty for Children with Postural Disorder

Poor Self-Esteem	Low self-esteem results from being teased mercilessly for being "slow" or "last" in physical education or at recess
	The child may be thought of as lazy, unmotivated, or "just doesn't care"
	The child may be so used to losing that he does not ever expect to succeed
	These problems can have a profound effect on his ability to learn and participate socially

Proprioceptive and Vestibular Issues	He often has weak muscles and a poor sense of where his body is in space
	He has difficulty resisting accidental bumps or nudges
	Being bumped may throw him off-balance and cause a fall
	Because of poor balance and weak muscles, he may be unable to dress himself, ride a bike, play tug-of-war, and participate in other games or activities that require muscle activation, pressure, or force
Poor Bilateral Coordination	He demonstrates poor bilateral coordination (using both sides of his body together)
	He has difficulty doing a task that requires two hands, such as rotating a piece of paper with one hand and cutting it with the other hand or holding a paper in place with one hand while writing on it with the other hand
	His lack of trunk rotation leads to difficulty with crossing the midline of his body to reach for objects or perform actions
	He has a tendency to use each hand independently—the right hand reaches for objects on his right side, and the left hand reaches for objects on his left side
Poor Ocular-Motor Control	He has difficulty with "smooth pursuits," such as using both eyes to follow an object that is moving in space
	He has difficulty smoothly moving his eyes across a line of print, as is required for reading
	He has other ocular-motor problems, such as poor convergence (using the eyes together), poor peripheral vision, and/or difficulty shifting his gaze quickly from the left to the right
	These impairments may require a referral to a developmental optometrist after an occupational therapist has sufficiently developed the stability of his core muscles in his trunk and neck

Principles of Intervention for Postural Disorder

A child with a postural disorder (like a child with sensory underresponsivity) often does not want to partake in motor activities. These two subtypes often co-occur. Children in both subtypes exhibit poor ocular-motor control, a poor ability to remain stable if pushed or pulled, weak muscles, and poor co-contraction. Almost always, a child with sensory underresponsivity will exhibit postural disorder. However, not all children with postural disorder have sensory underresponsivity.

In spite of some similar attributes, the subtypes are different in the manner in which sensory input is processed and in the responses that are made. Children with sensory underresponsivity are basically unaware of the sensory stimulation around them. Children with postural disorder know what is happening and what is expected of them; *they are aware,* but they cannot execute the required tasks, owing to a lack of stability in their trunk, poor rotation, a lack of muscle co-contracting, etcetera.

The key principles of intervention are provided as follows. In general, the overall goal is to increase the stability of the children's *core*—their trunk—when they move. Once they are more able to play like other children, the desired outcomes become increased social participation and self-confidence.

Principle 1: Boost the child's self-esteem.

This principle applies to all subtypes, as self-esteem is compromised in many children with SPD. However, this aspect of functioning is particularly noticeable in postural disorder. Many techniques exist for strengthening self-esteem and self-confidence. The main principle is that a child has to *try* a task that is hard for her, *and she must succeed,* and she must succeed, and then she must succeed again! To ensure that she succeeds, someone must *"scaffold"* the child in a given activity, or provide just enough help so the child does most of the activity on her own but receives whatever small boost she needs to finish successfully.

Lydia's Story

"I can't. I can't. I can't!" wailed Lydia, walking into the occupational therapy room for the first time. She looked at the zip line going into the ball pit, the swinging equipment, and the climber that looked like a jungle gym. "No way!" she said loudly, making sure everyone in the room could hear her.

"Okay," I said. "Let's just watch some of the kids having fun for today." Lydia looked at me suspiciously. "Okay," she said grumpily.

"Where do you want to sit?" I asked.

Lydia looked surprised. "Do I choose that?"

"Yes," I said. "In this room, everyone chooses what they want to do, and no one is forced to do anything."

Lydia looked confused. "But I thought I was here to work on things that are hard for me."

"Well," I said, "That's one reason you're here. But you don't exactly 'work' on things here. We only play here. And by playing just the right games, you will get better. By the way, is there anything you want to be better at?"

"I'm terrible at everything," Lydia replied.

"Well it seems to me that you are pretty good at talking," I said. "And also at telling people what you want and don't want. You'd be surprised how many kids can't do that."

"Really?" she said. "I never knew that."

"Here at the STAR Center, we like to know what kids can do really well and start there. What do you think you do really well?"

"Um…I dunno. I'm a real loser."

"Uh-huh," I murmured.

Then Lydia said softly, "But—well, I can sort of think up stories."

"Wow! That's cool," I said. "Can you show me how you do that?"

From that point in Lydia's first session, things got better. Our conversation took about 20 minutes, and her story took another 15 minutes, with her talking and me typing.

"This is a really cool story," I said. "Do you want me to print it out so you can make pictures to go with it at home?"

Lydia "won" what she wanted to do on that first day. Although (and because) she did what she wanted that day, on subsequent days we were able to work out a compromise so that she chose one activity, then I chose one activity. But all the activities we both chose were ones at which she succeeded (with or without assistance). It wasn't until we were well into her therapy time—about halfway through the set of 30 sessions—that Lydia trusted me enough to try things that were really hard for her. Luckily, she had parents who understood her need to control the sessions at first, and they trusted that I knew what I was doing.

It was interesting how Lydia never really talked about what she had done in therapy until the activities started getting hard, and yet despite the challenge, she was succeeding. Then she wanted her mom or dad to come watch her. It was yet another reminder that most children want to try challenging activities, but ones that are not so hard that they fail. And it was a poignant reminder of how your relationship with your child and her engagement with you *must* come before therapeutic activities. In Lydia's case, the problem was compounded by years of failing at tasks, being the last to be picked for the "teams" in P.E. class and at recess, and being teased by the other kids. Until she stopped beating herself up, until she knew that someone truly believed she *could* (and could *accurately judge* whether she *could* or not), until we collaborated—she would not have made progress.

Principle 2: Strengthen the child's "core" muscles.

Building strength in the child's abdominals and trunk muscles (which are often called *core muscles)* increases balance, improves posture, and helps with motor control and shifting weight from one side to the other. The core or "powerhouse" muscles include the abdominals, back, bottom, the muscles throughout the pelvic area, and the front and back of the upper legs (the quadriceps—called *quads* for short—and the hamstrings). The Noodle Kidoodle Movement Program helps strengthen the core muscles while a child moves from one movement pattern to another, working against gravity. This is one of the activities described in the next section, using A SECRET frame of reference.

Principle 3: Work in antigravity positions.

Antigravity positions are postures in which your body is moving against gravity. For example, if you lie on your stomach and raise your arms and legs up to "fly like an airplane," your body is having to lift against gravity. If you lie on your back and try to curl your head, shoulders, and legs up so that your whole body moves into a "little ball," you're having to lift up against gravity. We call any work that your body does that is against gravity an *antigravity position*.

It is crucial to start by having your child experience "safe" movements. When your child starts by lying on the floor, he or she will be less fearful. These floor positions ("airplane" and "little ball") can be hard work, and they get the child's proprioceptors and vestibular receptors used to working against gravity, while ensuring that the child feels comfortable and safe.

In the airplane position, the child lies on her stomach, arms held out straight in front of her body, with her legs extended straight out behind her. Holding this position for a few seconds (depending on the child's age) requires a great deal of control, works the core muscles that help her body to remain stable, and causes the muscles to co-contract (remember, *co-contracting* means that the muscles on the opposite sides of the body work equally, such as your biceps and your triceps. Isometric exercises are classic ways to acquire good co-contraction.)

As a child begins to master the easier positions on the floor, you can begin moving toward more challenging positions, such as having her lie over the top of a large therapy ball.

Principle 4: Use weight-bearing and resistive activities.

A *weight-bearing activity* is one in which parts of your body work with heavy weight on them. For example, if you were to climb a mountain with a heavy backpack, you would be weight-bearing—bearing or carrying extra weight. A *resistive* activity is one in which you resist a strong pull in a certain direction. For example, if you are arm-wrestling, and someone adds his power to your opponent's side, you would have to resist extra strength. When we use the term *resistive activity,* we are talking about adding some additional resistance (usually in the form of weight) to the effort that the child is making.

Activities that incorporate weight-bearing and resistance bring in additional proprioceptive input. This helps the child to develop a better sense of body awareness and comfort in knowing where her body is in space. A good way to do this and to teach parents to accomplish this is to play-wrestle with the child, allowing the child to move into a position in which you can provide some resistance. With younger children, you can have them try to push you over. Get on your hands and knees and have the child push against you. You could say something like, "You can huff and puff, but can you blow down this strong house?" (Of course, in the end, after providing excellent resistance, you allow the child to "blow you down!")

Now it's the child's turn. You say, "Okay, this time, don't let me knock you down! I'm going to huff and puff, so don't let me blow you over!" You must push just hard enough that the child's muscles contract, but not so hard that you push her down. When the child holds the position and remains still (as in isometric exercises), she must *co-contract* her muscles. Over time, this will increase her core stability (plus, it can be lots of fun!).

> ## Principle 5: For efficient upper-extremity function, work on developing stability across the shoulders, forearms, and wrists.

Stability of all the joints is important for function. For many children who have difficulty with fine-motor skills, stability of the joints and muscles of the arms and hands is needed. Good stability of the *upper extremities* can have a direct effect on school performance and self-help skills. Most people don't realize how important the shoulders and trunk are for good fine-motor ability. The arm, of course, starts at the shoulder, which is connected to the trunk. So if the trunk is weak, there is no way you can really improve a child's fine-motor skills without addressing trunk and shoulder stability first. (See chapter 10 on dyspraxia for more information about fine-motor planning.)

> ## Principle 6: Work on motor challenges as well as sensory difficulties.

Postural disorder and dyspraxia are not just about sensory challenges—they also affect motor difficulties. Therapists' goals are to build routines designed to help the child use *normal movement patterns* for as much of the day as possible. It is a bit technical and beyond the scope of this book to explain what a "normal movement pattern" is, exactly. However, if you suspect that your child has a postural disorder, try to get a therapist specially trained in neurodevelopmental therapy (you can ask your therapist if he or she has this background) so that your child's motor issues can also be addressed.

A SECRET for Children with Postural Disorder

As discussed in previous chapters, when you use A SECRET, you start by identifying the area of challenge that you want to pursue first. A child with postural disorder could potentially have challenges in a number of domains, including attention, sensation, and emotional regulation.

Imagine that we are working with Stewart, a 7-year-old with postural disorder. Stewart desperately wants to play volleyball with his friends. In spite of how hard this sport is for him, our job—whether we are his teacher, parent, or therapist—is to create strategies that will support Stewart in feeling good when he tries to meet the demands he will face during volleyball. (Just a side note here: Anything a child *really* wants to do is generally worth trying, because he will be so motivated!)

Let's begin by choosing a strategy to help address arousal and attention. We are going to use a movement activity to help Stewart "warm up" and increase his whole-body awareness through proprioceptive stimulation.

Activity 8A. Noodle Kidoodle Movement Program

Stewart is introduced to the Noodle Kidoodle Movement program, a fun set of activities that supports a child during transitional movements by using a swimming pool "noodle." This program encourages a child to move through a series of postures that start on the floor and gradually transition into an upright posture. The goal in using this particular movement program is to work the body as a whole and increase Stewart's endurance and tolerance to movement over time.

Stewart places the noodle behind his knees, feet, and back during the movement transitions. Postures are first done on the floor, where there is less pull from gravity, and then Stewart moves on to higher surfaces, which require greater postural demands. The noodle supports his body parts so Stewart feels secure while moving, stabilizing, and strengthening his core muscles.

In **Figure 8.3,** Laura holds the pool noodle while lying on the floor. Laura has very few postural demands in the first set of postures, as she is required to begin by lying on her back and then rolling onto her stomach. The noodle also provides some momentum during rolling. Laura and Stewart may feel challenged by this initially, as physically moving and "being moved" are scary.

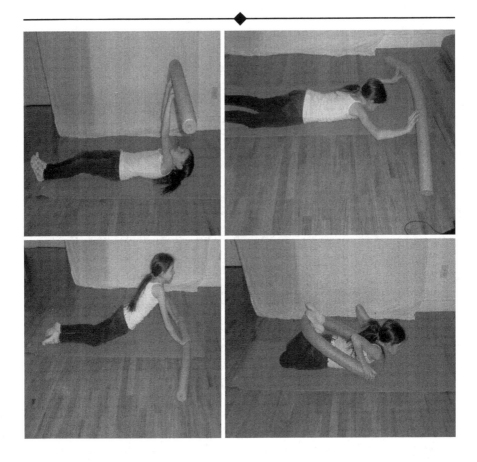

Figure 8.3. Laura demonstrates some positions with the pool noodle.

See the end of this chapter for details regarding the Noodle Kidoodle Movement Program and to see the additional postures that Laura gets into with ease and comfort while using the pool noodle.

Stewart will need a lot of support and encouragement in working toward feeling more comfortable moving in space. He needs emotional support and creative strategies that do not threaten him and that he can actually complete well. He is not used to taking risks that involve postural adjustments during dynamic, challenging motor tasks like playing volleyball. You could use emotional regulation to enhance his attention to the task.

Activity 8B. Vestibular Loading Exercises

This activity is called *vestibular loading*. It is a safe, supportive, and effective method to use the inner ear receptors, which stimulate the vestibular system. Here we are using sensation and emotional regulation to increase attention. This strategy can actually be used prior to Stewart going out to play volleyball, as it will help him to visually follow the ball and enhance his attention and arousal. Following these five steps constitutes the vestibular loading exercises:

1. Complete seven neck-rolls in one direction, and then repeat in the opposite direction.

2. Engage in head-and-neck nodding. First move your head and eyes up toward the ceiling seven times, then move your head and eyes down toward the floor seven times.

3. Turn your head from left to right, as if you're looking over your shoulder. Turn your head as far back as possible.

4. Tilt your ear toward your shoulder and hold the position to the count of three. Repeat, but tilt your opposite ear to your shoulder on the opposite side.

5. Place your hands behind you, clasped at your waist. Lean your body and head up toward the ceiling as far as you can go. Then lean your head and body down toward the floor as far as you can go. Complete both back-leaning and front-leaning five times each.

All of these exercises are designed to work in your natural planes, where vestibular receptors exist to detect and respond to changes in posture. Stewart may feel dizzy after completing the exercises. If so, he can press gently on his head with his clasped hands, so his neck proprioceptors can calm his "dizzies." We call this "pushing the dizzies out."

Activity 8C. Listen to Upbeat Music

Having fun is one of the most important aspects of strategies for all children with SPD. Stewart is not used to movement and feels awkward and uncomfortable when playing sports or doing other activities that involve movement. Listening to upbeat music helps keep everyone in a good mood during the *vestibular loading* exercises. Here we are using sensation and emotional regulation to increase attention.

When we use A SECRET, we are reminded to bring in so many important elements that are critical in helping a child feel more successful. Our approaches and plans are rich with strategies that not only support the specific challenged area that is interfering with the task, but also address relationships, emotional regulation, and culture. A SECRET will help you construct activities that are much more diverse and flexible and will ultimately meet the child's needs in a holistic manner. We have found that taking the time to regard all the elements of A SECRET creates a richness in intervention that is not ordinarily seen.

Activity 8D. Whole-Family Participation

This activity is aimed at changing the culture and relationships in Stewart's family by having all the kids practice volleyball together (relationship) *before* starting their homework (changing the *culture*). Here we are using the elements of culture and relationship simultaneously. Stewart's sister, brother, mom, and dad will join him in playing indoor volleyball with him in the basement, which has wall-to-wall carpeting and lots of padding. What a fun and safe place to practice before the "real game" is played!

Problem-Solve Using E = Environment: Support Stewart's Task Success

Stewart's family has changed the environment in their basement to clear a large section of the room so that the family can play volleyball there. By addressing the environment in the framework of A SECRET, we have thought through the changes needed to make the room comfortable and conducive for practice. We move the couch to the middle of the room and pretend it's a net. The family will use a small couch pillow in place of volleyball. (Later we'll discuss additional strategies for modifying the environment for children with postural disorder at school and at home.)

We have created some excellent strategies to support Stewart's issues in arousal and attention by using methods that incorporate sensation and movement, music, and vestibular loading exercises. We have addressed emotional regulation, cultural changes (by delaying homework until after family volleyball practice), and family involvement and support (aka *relationship*). Now let's take a final look at how to approach Stewart's desire to play volleyball to see if there are any other strategies that can be used to further support him.

Problem-Solve Using T = Task to Enhance Stewart's Attention

During the practice session the day before a game, let's actually bring in a volleyball to make it more real, just like it will be during the game. Instead of trying to hit the cushion over the couch, practice throwing and catching the ball first and then move toward volleying the ball.

Now let's address low-cost body stabilizers for children with postural disorder. Stabilizers will help improve upper-extremity function and skill for activities of daily living, sports, and other school-related tasks.

Cost-Effective Sitting Strategies in Postural Disorder

Remember how scared Barry felt during art class, when he was required to sit on a high stool with his feet off the ground? The poor stability he experienced throughout his core and pelvis made this class a "nightmare" for Barry.

Activity 8E. Using a Box for Pelvic Stability

Using a regular box to provide postural support is a simple, low-tech, and cost-effective strategy that can be implemented with younger children and toddlers through kindergarten. The box provides stability when a child sits in a chair or on a low stool that does not have back support.

The box you use should be snug and strong enough to help a child feel safe and secure. Cut one side of the box open so the child can sit directly inside, resembling a booster seat. The box provides stability in three dimensions: back, right, and left, as seen in **Figure 8.4.** Place the box on a chair or stool and line it with fabric to make it more comfortable. Make sure the chair is low enough that the child's knees are at about a 90° angle when he sits up straight. You can use a step stool or other aide to ensure that the child's feet rest on a high enough surface.

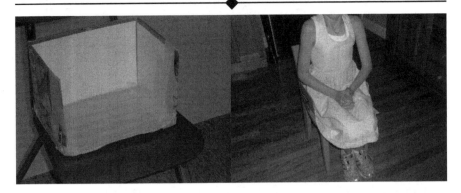

Figure 8.4. A box can be adapted so a
child can sit inside it for postural support.

Activity 8F. Use a Loose-Leaf Binder to Improve Pelvic Tilt

Children with poor *proximal stability* (core strength) tilt their pelvic area
significantly, which adds to their postural problems. They either tilt the pelvic
area forward, which creates a "C"-shaped spine, or tilt it backward, so their
shoulders move down toward their buttocks. Both postures interfere with
proper sitting alignment and contribute to difficulty in paying attention while
sitting in a chair. To add a feeling of comfort and stability and to train the pelvis
to move toward the proper position, you can place a 1-inch, hard, loose-leaf
binder inside the box.

The binder (which is an adaptation to the child's environment) resembles
the wedge that many therapists purchase commercially to correct alignment
of the child's pelvis in the chair. The goal in using the binder is to help the child
sit with a *neutral pelvis*, meaning that it is not tilted forward or backward.

When a child has a forward tilt in his pelvis (with his shoulders and hips
back and his stomach forward) **(Figure 8.5)**, place the binder so that the
taller side is in front (at the front of the box) **(Figure 8.6)**. This angle tips the
child's pelvis backward slightly to create a neutral position.

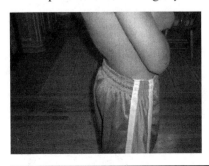

Figure 8.5. A boy's pelvis tilts forward.
When he sits, it will be helpful to get
him into a "neutral" position.

No Longer A SECRET

Sitting upright with a neutral pelvis enhances better attention and arousal states for learning.

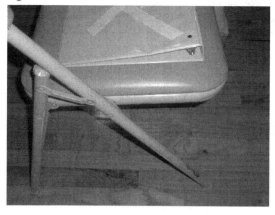

Figure 8.6. The taller side of the binder is placed in the front of the chair to correct a forward tilt.

If a child's pelvis is tipped toward the back, place the binder with the narrow side toward the front of the chair. This places his pelvis in a neutral position.

Table 8.2 gives you some more low-tech, affordable ideas to assist children with postural disorder.

Table 8.2. Additional Cost-Effective Activities for a Child with Postural Disorder

Sensory System	Activity
Proprioceptive	Wrap up in a blanket
	Roll down a steep hill
	Sleep in a sleeping bag
	Sit in a box in a chair
	Use pillows or comforters and lean on the elbows, knees, and hands (for weight-bearing)
	Kneel on small pieces of carpet while playing catch, doing yoga or Pilates, swimming, or doing animal walks, such as a hermit crab or bear walk

Visual/Ocular-Motor	Use visual-tracking charts to develop "smooth pursuits" (following a moving object with the eyes)
	Use flashlights in a darkened room to play "flashlight tag"
	Play tetherball, tennis, volleyball, or ping-pong or shoot a game of pool at a pool table
Bilateral Coordination	Catch a ball or beanbag, cut with scissors, make necklaces and jewelry out of macaroni and beads, etc
	Use "dressing dolls" to develop skills of self-care, buttoning, zipping, snapping, and tying shoelaces
Vestibular/Balance	Play hop-scotch, jump on and off low surfaces to begin with and increase the height, do step aerobics or martial arts, play "Twister," do motor mazes (creating a maze out of chairs, tables, pillows, etc)
	Do Wii activities that incorporate balance and quick postural changes, as in tennis, skiing, and bowling; use T-stools, balance boards, teeter-totters at the playground, and swings

Some children are just naturally comfortable moving around and actively exploring their surroundings. An 8-month-old baby feels secure and comfortable crawling over to an object that has rolled under a couch or has fallen on a chair. The baby will plan how to move her body and use other objects to help reach the top of the chair. She has a strong inner drive and a healthy curiosity that motivates her to figure out how things around her work.

Early on, children begin to develop order in their world through differentiating and discriminating among objects that are the same and/or different. Proprioception helps children become more efficient in crawling and developing balance and postural comfort so that ultimately, they will have the core strength to stand, run, jump, skip, climb, and further explore their environment. All of these skills are interdependent with postural control.

9

Sensory-based Motor Disorder—Dyspraxia

Dyspraxia is the second type of sensory-based motor disorder. Again, we'll show you how to use A SECRET to come up with helpful and meaningful strategies for children with dyspraxia. It's worth reiterating that when strategies are effective, a child feels successful and develops a sense of mastery, which is our ultimate goal for all the children with whom we work.

What Is Dyspraxia?

Essentially, dyspraxia is a motor-planning problem that occurs when a child has difficulty creating ideas for and executing motor action(s). Praxis (motor planning) is defined as the ability to think of, plan, sequence, and then execute new goal-directed actions. Praxis includes three distinct elements:

1. Cognitive visualizing or imagining an action (often called "ideation")

2. Planning and sequencing

3. Motor execution

Once a child learns how to do an activity automatically—without conscious thought—it no longer requires a motor plan. For example, when you are first learning to put on your clothes, it requires great concentration, and thus *praxis*. But when getting dressed becomes automatic at an older age, because planning is not required to get dressed automatically, it no longer taps into motor-planning abilities.

Think about a difficult motor task you learned to do recently. For me, it was learning how to roll a kayak in white water. I was taking a kayaking class with my daughter. Of course, at age 11, she simply turned upside down and rolled right back up as instructed. But me? No way! I rolled upside down, thought about all the things I was taught—flicking my hip, putting my arm out straight along the surface of the water, and pulling down and letting my trunk follow. Well, I turned upside down and my trunk followed right to the bottom of the pond as I came out of my kayak over and over. "Mom, you're thinking about it too much. Just do it! Like this..." Whoop! She went under. And whoop! She was upright again. It was a very humbling experience.

Can you remember learning to ride a bike? Initially, every step required effort and thought. You had to think about getting on the bike, sitting up tall on the seat, keeping your balance, putting your feet on the pedals, steering, and creating momentum for moving. After some trauma, bruises, and falling, riding became second nature and no longer required a motor plan. It is now an acquired skill that you have mastered and can execute automatically. (That is, until you try to ride a tandem bicycle with your husband...but that's another story!)

Children who have difficulty with motor planning often look clumsy and awkward and may become either self-conscious about their motor problems or, if self-assured, play the role of class clown.

There are three steps involved in the learning phase of motor planning:

1. Visualizing and/or creating a plan of action; in this case, knowing what riding a bike looks like and what you look like riding a bike, as well as knowing what you want to do with the bike.

2. Sequencing and organizing the steps involved in the plan of action (first you hold the handlebars, next you straddle the seat, etc).

3. Performing the action and riding the bike.

All three steps are of equal importance in the process of learning to ride a bike. After you've mastered the skill, however, you no longer have to think about it. You just get on and go. Riding is automatic. The need for a motor plan is gone.

Children with dyspraxia don't just have difficulty learning how to ride a bike. They struggle with far simpler tasks, such as getting dressed in the morning, placing books in a backpack, finding their way from one classroom to another, and many other daily activities. "I have no idea what to do!" are familiar words to parents who have children with dyspraxia.

In 1977, Dr A. Jean Ayres, the renowned occupational therapist who introduced the theory of sensory integration, gave a talk entitled, "What Does It Feel to Be Dyspraxic." She described the deep levels of frustration and challenge experienced in performing everyday routines. She indicated that dyspraxic children know what they want, but they but can't figure out how to do it. The environment simply "won't cooperate" for these children—it's the environment's fault. This leads to comments like, "The wall hit me," "The net won't hold still for me," or "It's someone else's fault." With dyspraxia, a child extends his difficulties to the social environment.

Symptoms and Behaviors of Dyspraxia

The following story illustrates the kind of frustration Ayres described. In this story, Steven's teacher, Ms Green, assigned her students a task that Steven doesn't have the planning skills or motor sequences to complete.

Steven's Story

Steven is a kindergartener who attends a regular public school in his local school district. It is project time, and he is sitting at a table with his classmates and a large container of clay. On the table, there are tools such as scissors, tongue depressors, and crayons. Steven's teacher, Ms Green, is excited about the project. She has received permission to use the kiln to fire the objects the children make, so they can be glazed and taken home to their mothers for Mother's Day. She says, "Now children, just use your imaginations—and make anything you want!"

The children squeal with glee and begin creating wonderful, imaginative objects out of the clay. Some of the children create animals, while others make buildings, cars, snowmen, and faces. All the kids are working busily, except for Steven, who sits staring at the clay.

Ms Green walks over and quietly asks if Steven needs help. "I don't know what to make," he tells her. He looks around the room and shrugs his shoulders. Ms Green knows that helping Steven visualize something familiar, something he might have made or done before, might spark an idea about what to make out of the clay.

Ms Green points to the clay and says, "Okay, how about making a clay sandwich? You know, like you do when you pack your lunch with your mom every morning." Steven gives her a half-smile and agrees that would be a good idea, but he continues to sit without taking any action.

Even with his teacher giving him the idea, Steven is still having a hard time initiating the sandwich idea, despite the fact that he helps his mom make his peanut butter and jelly sandwich every morning.

"What do I do first?" he asks. Ms Green patiently describes each step involved in making a sandwich. Steven listens, makes an effort toward beginning to make the sandwich, then looks up and says, "I got the first part—make a flat piece of 'bread.' But what do I do next?"

By now, Ms Green is losing her patience. Most of the other students have finished working with the clay and are starting to clean up. Steven just sits there, frustrated, and begins to cry. "I hate school!" he says.

Steven has poor planning and ideation. He can't sequence and organize the plan to make a sandwich, in spite of his real experience at home. Steven feels embarrassed, uttering under his breath that he's "just a stupid dumb-head." He wants to run away.

Teachers report that children with dyspraxia play with toys very differently than other children do. In the kindergarten block corner, all the boys are building elaborate projects with Lego blocks. Peter is having trouble putting the Lego pieces together in a meaningful pattern. He is watching the other boys whiz through their work effortlessly. He can't visualize how to begin the construction and is having difficulty fitting the small pieces inside one another. Peter gives up, frustrated. As he sits and watches the other boys build, he makes an impulsive decision to knock down their projects. At least someone will notice him. Now the boys are yelling at Peter and calling him "stupid," "idiot," and other derogatory names.

Across the room in the doll section, some girls are playing with Barbie dolls. Katy can't figure out how to put the clothes on the dolls and be part of the group. She glances over to where Christina and Lauren are putting really cool outfits on the Barbie dolls and feels frustrated. So, Katy gives up and just sits to the side, watching the others and sulking.

Both Peter and Katy feel really bad. They may even begin to equate their poor motor abilities with being unworthy. Children with dyspraxia need effective strategies to help them perform fine- and gross-motor skills at home and in the classroom. Strategies for improving fine-motor praxis are described at the end of this chapter.

The sensory components of dyspraxia and the correlated behaviors are noted in **Tables 9.1** and **9.2.**

Table 9.1. Effects of Poor Proprioceptive and Vestibular Processing (Movement-based Dyspraxia) on Motor Planning

Effects of Proprioceptive/Vestibular-based Problems	Has poor body awareness and difficulty organizing and planning movement sequences
	Demonstrates clumsy, awkward movements
	Has difficulty learning new motor tasks
	Has difficulty using new playground equipment
	Has difficulty finding her way around a new environment, including school hallways, friends' houses, and new playgrounds

Table 9.2. Effects of Poor Visual and Proprioceptive Processing on Gross- and Fine-Motor Skills and Lack of Coordination

Effects of Visual and Proprioceptive Problems	Demonstrates a poor ability to play team sports or create strategic moves that involve the use of timing and sequencing
	Has slow motor reactions and poor mental planning of movements
	Has difficulty with art projects, building, and putting small manipulative pieces together
	Has difficulty with fine-motor tasks, buttoning, tying shoelaces, zipping, using utensils, and typing
	Has difficulty writing legibly or learning to print or write in cursive

Robert's Story

Robert is playing in the gym. He is trying to jump over a moving pole. The pole is attached to a base that rotates and moves at various speeds. Robert is getting frustrated and falls over the pole. The demands placed on him during this task involve timing and sequencing that are just too hard for his current developmental level in motor functioning **(Figure 9.1)**. His actions don't match the required demands of the task. He trips and falls and quickly kicks the pole over. He is angry with the activity and with himself.

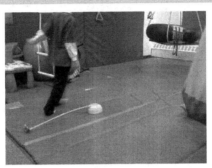

Figure 9.1. This child demonstrates poor timing and sequencing in jumping over the pole.

Table 9.3. Effects of Poor Tactile and Proprioceptive Processing (Difficulties in Fine-Motor and Self-Care Skills)

Effects of Tactile and Proprioceptive Challenges	Has difficulty with handwriting and learning cursive (graphomotor problems)
	Has difficulty acting out play schemes, setting up doll houses, dressing up, etc
	Has difficulty using classroom tools, scissors, and staplers, pasting, and doing construction-type activities
	Is a messy eater
	Has difficulty with dressing, undressing, and putting on stockings, tights, socks, mittens, and gloves; specifically, has difficulty putting arms into sleeves, legs into leg holes, and feet into the correct shoes
	Demonstrates poor fine-motor control, which influences the oral-motor musculature for regulation of drinking through a straw, chewing, blowing bubbles, and articulating speech

The primary subtypes of dyspraxia that Ayres identified were a vestibular-based motor-planning problem and a tactile/proprioceptive motor-planning problem. According to her research, the vestibular-based dyspraxic child usually had difficulty with bilateral coordination (using both sides of the body at the same time) and some academic tasks, such as math and reading, yet was able to almost self-treat, as he or she was generally of the subtype that seeks out stimulation. The tactile-proprioceptive–based dyspraxic child had significant body-based motor-planning issues that included poor body awareness, postural difficulties, and low endurance levels **(Table 9.3)**. Ocular-motor problems also occurred frequently. This is the classic dyspraxic profile that we often see in the clinic.

Note that the empirical data for subtypes of dyspraxia were developed by Ayres. This classification system needs further research before we will be confident in these subdivisions of dyspraxia. Nevertheless, from a treatment viewpoint, the classifications can help us target our intervention.

Principles of Intervention for Dyspraxia

This section provides general guidelines for working with any child who has dyspraxia. Incorporating the following principles will help organize motor-planning.

Principle 1: Work to boost the child's self-esteem.

Engaging and *relating* are the cornerstones of this treatment. A child really needs to trust you to be able to try tasks that are hard for him. You might consider starting with a familiar and favorite activity, perhaps one that the child can teach you. This approach will help him start on a positive note and not feel threatened about getting involved in play. By being asked to act the role of the teacher, he may begin to feel better about himself.

Principle 2: Sensory feedback enhances motor performance.

The more cues and proprioceptive feedback a child receives while performing an action, the more his body will feel the action, and the better his brain will remember how to perform it. Weights and resistant modalities, such as rubber bands and Ace bandages wrapped around the limbs (for short periods of time, maybe 20 minutes), are helpful forms of sensory input that enhance proprioception. When children develop a sense of their own bodies as they move, their performance improves.

Visual cues are another effective way to provide additional sensory input to enhance motor skills among dyspraxic kids. The visual input helps the child figure out a "plan" of how the action should look. One visual cue that most kindergarteners and first-graders find useful is a tiny picture of a proper pencil grip taped to their desk. The teacher can cue the children to check the picture when they're not holding their pencil correctly **(Figure 9.2)**.

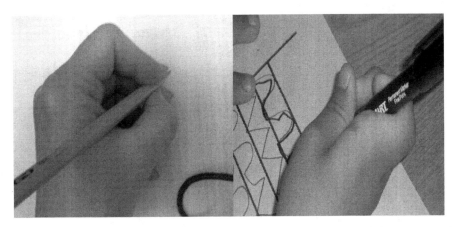

Figure 9.2. A depiction of an efficient grasp (on the left) versus an inefficient grasp (on the right).

A child with dyspraxia typically learns just one way to play a game. His or her rules, once learned, no longer require any thought or motor planning. When other children invent new rules—which they commonly do during play—the dyspraxic child may become very anxious and "quit" to avoid feeling incompetent. Show the child multiple things to do with objects and different ways to play games. Then, ask the child to think up even more ways to expand her ideas for each project you do together. She needs a lot of practice in thinking up new ideas; that way, she will be able join in play with children who tend to add to pretend-play games as they invent new characters, new crises, new locations, and the like.

It's crucial to realize that a child with dyspraxia often learns "splinter skills" (compensatory skills). For example, if she has learned to catch a softball, she may still feel challenged in kickball, volleyball, and soccer, because all of these sports involve different motor plans. The skills learned in softball do not necessarily transfer over like they do for typically developing children.

Principle 3: Encourage activities that require specific motions of the body in space.

Dynamic motor tasks like jumping, climbing, and hopping should be practiced with a child who has dyspraxia. Playing "Simon Says," using only verbal directions, requires a child to think about his or her body and make postural responses to verbal commands. Bring directionality and spatial elements into the instructions, such as, "Simon says put your right hand on your left knee and your left hand on your right ear." Spatial mapping is required to succeed in this task. A child who moves comfortably is using proprioception to assist in this action.

Principle 4: Choose activities that include elements of timing and sequencing.

Motor actions require a progression and order in which the actions are performed. You can't put your feet into the stirrups before you get up on the horse. Verbal and visual labeling of the required sequence of steps may be helpful for a child with dyspraxia. The more you can verbalize (or better yet, provide a picture of) the necessary sequence ahead of time (or the ongoing sequence during an activity), the better practice a child will get for one of the three important elements of praxis. When you think about it, every daily activity requires some degree of sequencing. One activity that will save you a lot of time in the morning is to have your child lay out his clothes on the bedroom floor the night before, so that the clothes are situated in the order needed (underwear, pants, shirt) for the morning.

Principle 5: Teach your child the goal of the activity.

As your child gets better at conceptualizing plans, goals of activities will be understood more easily. In using the baseball game example, you might explain to your child that, "In baseball, the winner is the team that gets the most home runs." You can use a visual picture of a baseball field and show your child how a home run is scored. Teach your child the steps involved—the sequences required to reach the goal.

Let your child create visual schedules to plan the day and the week's events. Visual schedules, particularly when written on a weekly calendar, help provide him with an overall picture of the activities he will be involved in.

▶ Principle 6: Practice mapping where you are and where you are going.

Most children with dyspraxia have difficulty locating themselves in space. Mapping can be a useful tool. Start with easier things like, "Let's draw a picture (or map) of where things are in your bedroom." Move up to mapping rooms in your house and then your house on your street. Try mapping the route to school or to a park. These activities will help give your child a picture of where he is located.

▶ Principle 7: Practice ideation (day in and day out).

Ideation is having ideas. Instead of always telling your child what to do, give him two choices and ask him, "Which one do you want to do?" "Do you want to use the red plate or the blue plate?" "Should we fill up the gas in the car now or after going shopping?" "In what order do you think we should do homework, a snack, and sensory breaks this afternoon?"

The best ideation tasks are ones where you do not supply *any* choices. For example, "I saw this box of popsicle sticks. Let's make things. What can we make?" Or, it could be building with snow or making sand castles—there are so many opportunities for your child to practice having ideas. Let him try.

A SECRET for Dyspraxia

Children with dyspraxia have many motor challenges that interfere with success in required tasks at home and at school. School frequently calls for much higher-level demands than the developmental abilities of children with motor-planning issues. By kindergarten, children are typically expected to write, copy, draw, and cut with scissors. Homework is often given to review and reinforce concepts presented during the school day. Thus, parents, after a hard day of work, are often expected to work with their children in the evenings to do homework, which can be frustrating for everyone in the family.

As kids get older and the gap widens between what they can do and what their peers can do, your child may become sullen and prone to giving up. Another problem is that many children with dyspraxia are quite intelligent, and the gap between their cognitive skills and their motor abilities may place them in "less advanced groups," just because they can't do the written work required to be in the "more advanced groups." It's a terrible tragedy that can lead to mental health issues and eventual trouble in the juvenile justice system.

Let's use A SECRET framework to problem-solve for how we can help Elizabeth, a dyspraxic child, feel more successful when completing a diorama that entails the use of a lot of fine-motor skills. Here are some typical instructions for making a diorama that any child might receive at school (we got ours from *www.wikihow.com*):

1. *Choose a habitat to create for your diorama.* Make sketches of how you want your diorama to look as you plan the front, back, sides, and top. Make the inside of the diorama look as deep and as three-dimensional as you can. Make a list of the things you will need to make your diorama. Use a variety of materials.

   Already, Elizabeth is in trouble. Are you kidding? Sketch the front, back, sides, and top?

2. *Make a base for the model out of a shoebox* or other box about the size of a shoebox. Find small figures to go along with your scene or make them out of clay, printouts, pipe cleaners, plasticine, or other materials. Use your imagination—it is the best art tool!

   "Oh sure, make figures out of plasticine," Elizabeth thinks. Note: Children with dyspraxia feel like they have mittens on when they are working with their hands.

3. *Be creative.* Anything you can find (cotton balls, leaves, twigs, etc) will usually work. Make every detail count.

   Creativity isn't Elizabeth's problem. However, sticking cotton balls and twigs in small places just isn't going to happen.

4. *Hang flying objects with clear string, such as monofilament used for fishing line,* if you have it. If you don't, ribbon that's the same color as the background will work, as well. Make sure you keep the lid of the box to cover up your work. You don't want it to get ruined!

   "You've got to be kidding!" thinks Elizabeth. "Flying objects hanging from monofilament? And the teacher said this was one homework project we'd all like. Guess what? She doesn't even know me or care about what I can and can't do."

So what's Elizabeth going to do now?

Problem-Solve Using Sequencing of Motor Activities to Enhance Attention

Elizabeth, like all children with dyspraxia, comes home from school exhausted. She's been required to *keep it together* all day long. The last thing Elizabeth wants to deal with is making a diorama. Rather then get right down to homework—which is a typical routine in many families—let's do a fun activity instead. You think, "A sensory preparation activity will get her nervous system into the right mode before doing homework. Purposeful, sequential motor activities will help Elizabeth feel more organized."

Make pictures of simple gross-motor activities on index cards (such as rolling, jumping, and hopping). Elizabeth gets to set the cards up in the sequence that she wants **(Figure 9.3).** The sequence is the order in which the actions will be performed. Elizabeth can set up and perform multiple motor chains before doing the final step in this game, which is starting the diorama. See if applying sensation through movement—including laughing and playing with you as you also complete the motor chain—helps Elizabeth get ready to sit down and work. (Doing obstacle courses or jumping on trampolines can also help increase attention and arousal for dyspraxic kids.)

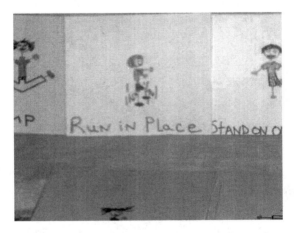

Figure 9.3. Sequences of motor moves can be used to enhance attention.

The diorama requires a lot of writing. When Elizabeth imagines the page she needs to write for the diorama, her eyes get watery and her smile turns into a pout. Writing is so very hard for her.

We have addressed some whole-body work in doing the gross-motor activities in the motor chain game. Let's use the element of sensation again and help Elizabeth use her fine-motor muscles to prepare for writing.

Problem-Solve Using Tactile and Proprioceptive Loaded Activities to Enhance Sensation

Introduce writing activities by using clothespins or chopsticks to pick up small items before attempting to write. Both of these items provide sensory feedback to the fingers about what they're doing. Through muscle memory, these exercises will help Elizabeth adjust her finger pressure when writing and coloring. **Figure 9.4** depicts the use of a clothespin and modified chopsticks, which are separated by a rolled-up piece of paper and fastened with a rubber band.

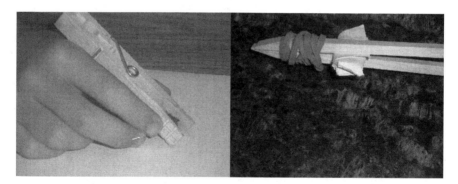

Figure 9.4. Use a clothespin or modified chopsticks to help develop a proper grasp for writing.

Part of Elizabeth's anxiety about doing homework stems from a lack of confidence due to constant teasing and rejection from her peers. It's important to help her feel better about herself so she can muster her inner drive and begin making her diorama. The element of emotional regulation will help with her self-esteem.

Sit down with Elizabeth and let her tell you what her homework is all about. This can be a short, 5-minute activity that will give her the opportunity to verbally organize her thoughts about the diorama. Elizabeth is acting out the role of teacher for a few minutes. She is explaining to you what needs to be done. So you're tackling two things at once—helping her gain confidence through emotional regulation and encouraging her to come up with a plan for her homework project.

Actually, this strategy incorporates more than just emotional regulation. It marks a change in the typical culture of how homework is approached in your home, now that you understand Elizabeth's dyspraxia better. You used to sit down with Elizabeth and tell her what she needed to do for homework. Now the roles have been switched by tweaking the culture at home. You and Elizabeth are spending quality time together, bonding over homework, of all things! What used to be a source of stress in your house has brought you closer and helped boost your daughter's self-esteem.

Just a quick reminder: Relationships are the most important element in A SECRET framework. Children who trust their parents, teachers, therapists, and friends go a lot further in their efforts on specific tasks—and probably in life—than kids who do not have a foundation of solid relationships.

You can help Elizabeth by creating a visual schedule for her project, with pictures or words that outline a specific plan. This will help her visualize the sequence in which things need to get done. The act of making the homework plan—not just taking the steps for the steps' sake—will be helpful in getting her started **(Figure 9.5)**.

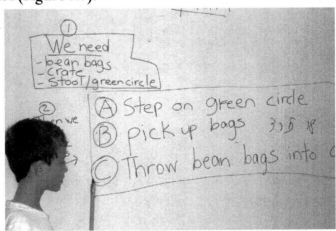

Figure 9.5. Developing a visual schedule or plan.

Talk about where the diorama will be made. In the kitchen? At her desk in her room? Allow Elizabeth to visualize and prepare the environment that is best for her. Self-advocacy is critical for children to become independent. Elizabeth goes to her room and brings out the shoebox that her hiking boots came in. Instead of making figurines, she decides to use a few of the Disney characters she collects. She starts to write down her plan, using a special technique she learned at school. She inclines her loose-leaf notebook to position her paper and wrist at a better angle for holding a pencil and uses an efficient grasp. Next, we see that Elizabeth has turned her chair sideways as she slides it alongside the table. She remembers the Chair Moves strategy that was taught to her class (Chair Moves positions 2 and 3 in chapter 6). She unwraps the lollipop that you have placed on the table for her, puts it into her mouth, and starts her homework. "Mom, can you put Mozart on while I write?" she asks. Elizabeth has successfully come up with strategies that address her environment and task. She has learned so much and benefited from the strategies you've incorporated to help her achieve success.

Finally, Elizabeth is ready to do her homework and is in a positive, *"calm-alert"* readiness state. This is going to be a very difficult project for Elizabeth. We recommend that you decide together what is a reasonable duration of time for her to work on it independently and that perhaps you buddy with her afterward to complete the project. After all, the project is not designed to evaluate fine-motor skills. As long as the creative ideas come from Elizabeth, it doesn't hurt to give her a little help.

One other tip about hand-written homework: Not everyone agrees with us, but we feel strongly that intelligent children who have severe handwriting problems should be taught typing skills as early as possible. Yes, it is important to write, but we feel that excessive time spent on handwriting exercises might sometimes be better spent on creative tasks or, say, reading. We recommend an early introduction to typing so that children can get their thoughts out, whether or not they have fine-motor problems.

Table 9.4 presents some additional cost-effective ideas to assist children with dyspraxia.

Table 9.4. Additional Cost-Effective Sensory Activities for Children with Dyspraxia

Sensory Input	Activity
Vestibular/ Proprioceptive/Visual	Motor mazes
	Tae kwon do
	Karate
	Kickboxing
	Martial arts
	Fun zones (ball pits, giant slides, etc)
	Dancing while singing; karaoke
	Following simple choreography
	Twister
	Jumping into target areas
	Trampolines
	Ice-skating and roller-skating
	Skiing
Oral-Motor Praxis	Blow toys
	Bubbles
	Blowing instruments: harmonicas, horns, blow-paint art

Tactile/ Proprioceptive/Visual	Baking, following a recipe
	Games like Mouse Trap and Operation
	Textured pop beads
	Theraputty; various colors for different resistances
	Barrel of Monkeys
	Pick-Up Stix
	Don't Break the Ice
	Ants in the Pants
	Mr. Mouth
	Hungry Hungry Hippos
	Etch-a-Sketch
	Miniature pool tables
	Table hockey
	Bowling
	Copper tooling
	Pipe-cleaner activities
	Wikki Stix
	Timers
	Charts
	Watches that provide sensory input, like vibration, to help a child with temporal and spatial difficulties
	Using color, a great visual cue for labeling and helping a child sequence events
	Whack-a-Mole
	Simon
	Throwing games (as at a target)
	Tracing and drawing
	Dot-to-dot games and fine-motor coordination activities
	Weaving activities
	Parquetry (geometric) pattern cards and blocks
	Lacing activities
	Sticker art

References

1. Miller LJ, Coll JR, Schoen SA. A randomized controlled pilot study of the effectiveness of occupational therapy for children with sensory modulation disorder. *Am J Occup Ther*. 2007;61(2):228-238.

2. Miller LJ, Anzalone ME, Lane SJ, Cermak SA, Osten ET. Concept evolution in sensory integration: a proposed nosology for diagnosis. *Am J Occup Ther*. 2007;61(2):135-140.

3. McIntosh DN, Miller LJ, Shyu V, Hagerman RJ. Sensory-modulation disruption, electrodermal responses, and functional behaviors. *Dev Med Child Neurol*. 1999;41(9):608-615.

4. Cross KP. *Collaborative Learning Techniques: A Handbook for College Faculty*. San Francisco, CA: Josse-Bass; 2005.

5. Cameron OG. Interoception: the inside story—a model for psychosomatic processes. *Psychosom Med*. 2001; 63(5):697-710.

6. Miller LJ, Cermak S, Lane S, Anazalone M, Koomar J. Defining sensory processing disorder and its subtypes: position statement on terminology related to sensory integration dysfunction. *SI Focus*. Summer 2004:6–8.

7. Miller LJ, Lane SJ, Cermak SA, Anzalone M, Osten B. Regulatory-sensory processing disorders in children. In: Greenspan SI, Wieder S, eds. *Diagnostic Manual for Infancy and Early Childhood: Mental Health, Developmental, Regulatory-Sensory Processing, Language and Learning Disorders*. Bethesda, MD: Interdisciplinary Council on Developmental and Learning Disorders; 2005:73-112.

8. Miller LJ. *Sensational Kids: Hope and Help for Children with Sensory Processing Disorder*. New York, NY: Penguin Group; 2006.

9. James K, Miller LJ, Schaaf R, Nielsen DM, Schoen SA. Phenotypes within sensory modulation dysfunction. http://www.elsevier.com/wps/find/journaldescription.cws_home/623360/description. *Compr Psychiatry*. Published February 8, 2001. Accessed May 19, 2011.

10. Ahn R, Miller LJ, Milberger S, McIntosh DN. Prevalence of parents' perceptions of sensory processing disorders among kindergarten children. *Am J Occup Ther.* 2004;58(3):287-302.

11. Ben-Sasson A, Carter AS, Briggs-Gowan MJ. Sensory over-responsivity in elementary school: prevalence and social-emotional correlates. *J Abnorm Child Psychol.* 2009;37:705–716.

12. Goldsmith HH, Van Hulle CA, Arneson CL, Schreiber JE, Gernsbacher MA. A population-based twin study of parentally reported tactile and auditory defensiveness in young children. *J Abnorm Child Psychol.* 2006;34(3):393–407.

13. May-Benson TA, Koomar JA, Teasdale A. Incidence of pre-, peri-, and post-natal birth and developmental problems of children with sensory processing disorder and children with autism spectrum disorder. *Frontiers Integrative Neurosci.* 2009;3(31):1-12.

14. Schneider ML, Moore CF, Gajewski LL, et al. Sensory processing disorder in a primate model: evidence from a longitudinal study of prenatal alcohol and prenatal stress effects. *Child Dev.* 2008;79(1):100-113.

15. Miller LJ. *Sensational Kids: Hope and Help for Children with Sensory Processing Disorder.* New York, NY: Penguin Group; 2006.

16. Eisenberg N, Hofer C, Vaughan J. Effortful control and its socioemotional consequences. In: Gross JJ, ed. *Handbook of Emotion Regulation.* New York, NY: Guilford Press; 2007:287-306.

17. Shonkoff JP, Phillips DA. *From Neurons to Neighbourhoods: The Science of Early Childhood Development.* Washington, DC: National Academy Press; 2000.

18. Lewit EM, Baker LS. School readiness. *Future Child.* 1995;5(2):128-139.

19. Blair C, Razza RP. Relating effortful control, executive function, and false belief understanding to emerging math and literacy ability in kindergarten. *Child Dev.* 2007;78(2):647-663.

20. Johnson DJ, Jaeger E, Randolph SM, Cauce AM, Ward J, and the NICHD Early Child Care Research Network. Studying the effects of early child care experiences on the development of children of color in the United States: Toward a more inclusive research agenda. *Child Dev.* 2003;74(5):1227-1244.

21. Blair C, Razza RP. Relating effortful control, executive function, and false belief understanding to emerging math and literacy ability in kindergarten. *Child Dev.* 2007;78(2):647-663.

22. Shoda Y, Mischel W, Peake PK. Preschool delay of gratification: Identifying diagnostic conditions. *Dev Psychol.* 1990;26:978-986.

23. Williams B R, Ponesse JS, Schachar RJ, Logan G.D, Tannock R. Development of inhibitory control across the life-span. *Dev Psychol.* 1999;35:205–213.

24. Eisenberg N, Cumberland A, Spinrad TL. Parental socialization of emotion. *Psychol Inq.* 1998;9(4):241-273.

25. Gross JJ. Antecedent- and response-focused emotion regulation: divergent consequences for experience, expression, and physiology. *J Pers Soc Psychol.* 1998;74(1):224-237.

26. Lindberg JA, Swick AM. Common-sense classroom management: surviving September and beyond in the elementary classroom. Thousand Oaks, CA: Corwin Press, 2002.

27. Walker M. *The Power of Color.* New York, NY: Avery Publishing Group; 1991.

28. Jin EW, Shevell SK. Color memory and color constancy. *J Opt Soc Am A Opt Image Sci Vis.* 1996;13(10):1981-1991.

29. Radeloff DJ. Role of color in perception of attractiveness. *Percept Motor Skills.* 1990;71(1):151-160.

30. Underhill P. *Why We Buy: The Science of Shopping.* New York, NY: Simon and Schuster; 2000.

31. Bornstein BH, Neely CB, LeCompte DC. Visual distinctiveness can enhance recency effects. *Mem Cognit.* 1995;23(3):273-278.

32. Terwogt MM, Hoeksma JB. Colors and emotions: preferences and combinations. *J Gen Psychol.* 1995;122(1):5-17.

33. Johnson K. The effects of six colors on teenage mood states. *KJ*Research.* 1998. www.inmind.com/schools/CVGS/sturesearch/Johnson/.

34. Law MB, Pratt J, Abrams RA. Color-based inhibition of return. *Percept Psychophys.* 1995;57(3):402-408.

35. Chudler EH. Neuroscience for Kids. http://faculty.washington.edu/chudler/neurok.html. Accessed May 19, 2011.

36. McIntosh DN, Miller LJ, Shyu V, Hagerman RJ. Sensory-modulation disruption, electrodermal responses, and functional behaviors. *Dev Med*

Child Neurol. 1999;41(9):608-615.

37. Dunn W, Brown C. Factor analysis on the Sensory Profile from a national sample of children without disabilities. *Am J Occup Ther.* 1997;51(7):490-495.

38. James K, Miller LJ, Schaaf R, Nielsen DM, Schoen SA. Phenotypes within sensory modulation dysfunction. http://www.elsevier.com/wps/find/journaldescription.cws_home/623360/description. *Compr Psychiatry.* Published February 8, 2001. Accessed May 19, 2011.

39. Dunn W. The sensations of everyday life: empirical, theoretical and pragmatic considerations. *Am J Occup Ther.* 2001;55(6):608-620.

40. Ahn RR, Miller LJ, Milberger S, McIntosh DN. Prevalence of parents' perceptions of sensory processing disorders among kindergarten children. *Am J Occup Ther.* 2004;58(3):287-293.

41. Ognibene TC. *Distinguishing sensory modulation dysfunction from attention-deficit/hyperactivity disorder: sensory habituation and response inhibition processes* [dissertation]. Denver, Colorado: University of Denver; 2002.

42. Burleigh JM, McInstosh KW, Thompson MW. Central auditory processing disorders. In: *Sensory Integration Theory and Practice.* 2nd ed. Bundy A, Lane SJ, Murray E, eds. Philadelphia, PA: F.A. Davis, Co; 2001:141-165.

Resources

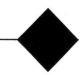

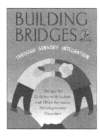

Paula Aquilla, Ellen Yack, & Shirley Sutton
*Building Bridges through Sensory Integration,
2nd edition*
www.sensoryworld.com

Britt Collins, MS, OTR/L, & Jackie Olson
*Sensory Parenting: From Newborns to Toddlers—
Everything Is Easier When
Your Child's Senses Are Happy!*
www.sensoryworld.com

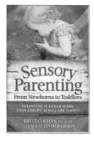

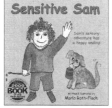

Marla Roth-Fisch
Sensitive Sam: Sam's sensory adventure has a happy ending!
www.sensoryworld.com

Dr Temple Grandin
The Way I See It: A Personal Look at Autism & Asperger's
www.fhautism.com

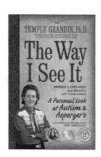

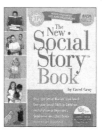

Carol Gray
The New Social Story Book
www.fhautism.com

Jennie Harding
*Ellie Bean, the Drama Queen: How Ellie Learned to Keep Calm
and Not Overreact!*
www.sensoryworld.com

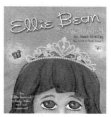

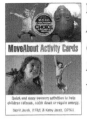

David Jereb, OTR/L, & Kathy Koehler Jereb, LOTA
MoveAbout Activity Cards:
Quick and Easy Sensory Activities to Help Children Refocus, Calm
Down or Regain Energy
www.sensoryworld.com

Joan Krzyzanowski, Patricia Angermeier,
& Kristina Keller Moir
Learning in Motion: 101+ Fun Classroom Activities
www.sensoryworld.com

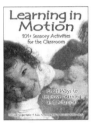

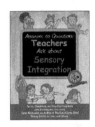

Jane Koomar, Stacey Szklut, Carol Kranowitz, et al
Answers to Questions Teachers Ask about Sensory Integration
www.sensoryworld.com

Aubrey Lande, MS, OTR, & Bob Wiz, Lois Hickman,
et al
Songames^{TM} for Sensory Processing (CD)
www.sensoryworld.com

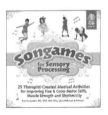

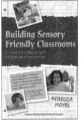

Rebecca Moyes
Building Sensory Friendly Classrooms
to Support Children with Challenging Behaviors
www.sensoryworld.com

Laurie Renke, Jake Renke, & Max Renke
I Like Birthdays...It's the Parties I'm Not Sure About!
www.sensoryworld.com

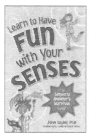

John Taylor, PhD
Learn to Have Fun with Your Senses!
The Sensory Avoider's Survival Guide
www.sensoryworld.com

Kelly Tilley, MS, OTR/L
Active Imagination Activity Book:
50 Sensorimotor Activities to Improve
Focus, Attention, Strength, & Coordination
www.sensoryworld.com

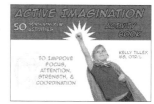

Carol Kranowitz, MA
The Out-of-Sync Child, 2nd ed;
The Out-of-Sync Child Has Fun, 2nd ed;
Getting Kids in Sync (DVD featuring the children of St. Columba's Nursery
    School);
Growing an In-Sync Child;
Sensory Issues in Learning & Behavior (DVD);
The Goodenoughs Get in Sync;
Preschool Sensory Scan for Educators (Preschool SENSE) Manual and Forms
    Packet

www.sensoryworld.com

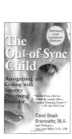
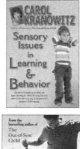
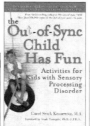
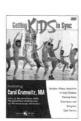
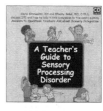
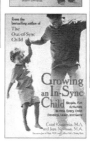

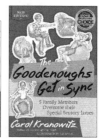

Online Resourses

www.sinetwork.org

www.spdfoundation.net

www.spdparentsupport.com

www.sensory-processing-disorder.com

www.spdlife.org

www.sensoryworld.com

www.spdsupport.org

www.spdbloggernetwork.com

About the Authors

Doreit S. Bialer

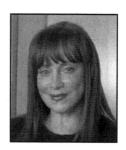

Doreit S. Bialer, MA, OTR/L, is a nationally recognized keystone speaker with more than 15 years of experience in pediatrics. She received an advanced master's degree in occupational therapy from New York University and is pursuing her doctorate in occupational therapy (pediatric science) at Rocky Mountain University in Utah.

Doreit co-owns a large private practice in Long Island, New York, where she works with children of all ages. In addition, she is an independent contractor to school districts in Nassau County, New York.

Doreit holds a number of certifications in neurodevelopmental therapy for both children and adults, as well as in the administration and interpretation of praxis tests. She is certified to use the Integrated Listening System and the Interactive Metronome, holds a personal-training degree with the Academy of Applied Personal Training Education (AAPTE), and is a certified Pilates Mat Instructor. Her background includes studies in anatomy and physiology of human performance, resistive-training biomechanics, health and fitness assessments, and basic nutrition. She has developed programs in vestibular rehabilitation for both adult and pediatric populations, with contributions from New York University Hospital and otolaryngologists.

Doreit teaches at the university level, including coursework in pediatrics, neuroanatomy, and kinesiology. She is an instructor for Summit Professional Education and the Bureau of Education and Research. Her national seminars focus on current strategies for occupational therapists who work in schools and on multisensory tools and techniques for children with SPD. Her newest endeavors include the development of a therapeutic Pilates course for children with sensorimotor challenges.

Lucy Jane Miller

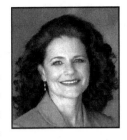

Dr Lucy Jane Miller founded the first comprehensive SPD research program in the nation and authored the groundbreaking book, *Sensational Kids: Hope and Help for Children with Sensory Processing Disorder*. She has been investigating, analyzing, and explaining SPD to other scientists, professionals, and parents since she studied under sensory-integration pioneer A. Jean Ayres more than 30 years ago. Since then, studies by Dr Miller and her colleagues have helped bring SPD widespread recognition, and her work with families has improved countless lives. Thanks to Dr Miller's mobilization of the research community, SPD now appears in two diagnostic manuals: the *Diagnostic Manual for Infancy and Early Childhood* and *The Diagnostic Classification: Zero to Three*. She has been working tirelessly to have SPD included in the 2013 revision of the *Diagnostic and Statistical Manual of Mental Disorders*. Dr Miller has also developed seven nationally standardized tests for use worldwide to assess and diagnose SPD and other developmental disorders and delays. Her widespread recognition and enormous credibility within the professional community are part of the reason that advanced clinicians travel from all over the world to be mentored by Dr Miller and her team at the SPD Foundation.

The prominence of Dr Miller's research, her compassion for and connection with "sensational" families, and her ability to explain the science of SPD clearly and empathetically make her a natural interview target. She has been featured on NBC's "Today Show" and ABC's "20/20," as well as in *The New York Times* and numerous other popular and professional publications. She is the author of more than 60 articles and/or chapters in scientific and professional journals, magazines, and textbooks and is a frequent presenter and speaker at conferences and workshops worldwide. She has received more than 30 funded awards and grants to further research on SPD and other childhood disabilities.

In 2004, Dr Miller received the Award of Merit from the American Occupational Therapy Association, which is the profession's highest honor and is reserved for therapists who have made an outstanding global contribution to the field. In 2005, she was awarded the Martin Luther King Jr Humanitarian Award by the state of Colorado for her three decades of work with children who have SPD.

Index

An **f** denotes a figure; a **t**, a table.

 A

B

C

D

E

F

G

system, 22

underresponsivity, 113–114, 113f

"Heavy work," 82, 135

Homeostasis, 56

Individual differences, 26, 35

Interoceptive domain

    overresponsivity, 79, 80t

    sensory discrimination disorder, 162, 162t

    system, 25–26

    underresponsivity, 106t

Key Ring Game, 63, 63f

Linking activities to emotional states, 62, 62f

Motivating activities, 109–110

Music for

    emotional regulation, 46

overresponsivity, 84

postural disorder, 191–192

sensory discrimination, 158

underresponsivity, 107, 111, 121

Occupational therapists, 18–19

Olfactory system, 22

Overresponsivity

auditory, 76, 76t

characteristics of, 71

definition, 74–75

fuel tank analogy applied to, 72–73, 72f

interoceptive, 79, 80t

as sensory modulation disorder, 29

symptoms and behaviors in, overview, 75

tactile, 76, 77t

taste and smell, 78, 78t

vestibular, 78–79, 79t

Overresponsivity, principles of intervention for

activity suggestions, 99–102

A SECRET activities, 96–98

avoidance of overstimulating sensory events, 83

calm responses to, 82

compression jacket, 89–90, 90f

conditions, 91t, 92

emotional regulation, 91t, 92

environment, 93, 93t, 94f, 94–95

P

Predictability, 81–82

Pretend play for emotional regulation, 57–58

Problem-solving process, 37, 41, 42t

Proprioceptive

    dyspraxia, 201t, 202t

    sensory discrimination disorder, 154–156, 155t

    system, 24–25

    underresponsivity, 107t

R

Relationships, 48, 49t

Rewards vs punishment, 58

S

Self-awareness survey, 67–68

Self-regulation, 84–85

Sensation, 43, 44t, 45

Sensational Kids: Hope and Help for Children with Sensory Processing Disorder, 40

Sensory backpacks, 83, 84f, 89

Sensory-based motor disorder

    dyspraxia, 31–32

    postural, 31

    sensory discrimination, 32–33

Sensory diet, problems with, 55–56

Sensory discrimination disorder

    definition, 151

    gustatory, 161, 161t

subtypes. *See* Subtypes, Sensory Processing Disorder

Sensory systems

auditory, 21

gustatory, 22

interoceptive, 25–26

olfactory, 22

overview, 20–21

proprioceptive, 24–25

tactile, 22–23

vestibular, 23–24

visual, 21–22

Sensory underresponsivity. *See* Underresponsivity

SPD. *See* Sensory Processing Disorder (SPD)

Stoplight Bracelet Game, 59–60, 59f, 60f

Subtypes, Sensory Processing Disorder

combinations of, 35, 36t, 38t, 39

controversy about, 26–27

diagnostic usefulness of, 27–28

sensory discrimination disorder, 33

overview, 28f

sensory-based motor disorder, 31–33

sensory modulation disorder, 29–31

T

Tactile domain

dyspraxia, 202t

overresponsivity, 76, 77t

sensory discrimination disorder, 154, 154t

❦ *U* ❦

---

music, 107, 111, 121

stimulation of taste and smell, 108–109, 109f

whole-body responses, 107–108, 108f

Vestibular domain

dyspraxia, 201t

overresponsivity, 78–79, 79t

sensory discrimination disorder, 160, 160t

system, 23–24

underresponsivity, 106t

Visual domain

dyspraxia, 201t

overresponsivity, 77, 77t

sensory discrimination disorder, 156, 157t

system, 21–22

underresponsivity, 105t

Weighted items

and emotional regulation, 55

and overresponsivity, 87t, 88